SEEDS OF MORTALITY

SEEDS OF MORTALITY

The Public and Private Worlds of Cancer

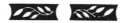

STEWART JUSTMAN

CHICAGO *Ivan R. Dee* 2003

Library of Congress Cataloging-in-Publication Data:
Justman, Stewart.
    Seeds of mortality : the public and private worlds of cancer / Stewart Justman.
        p. cm.
    Includes bibliographical references and index.
        ISBN 1-56663-498-9 (alk. paper)
        1. Cancer—Social aspects. 2. Rhetoric. 3. Prostate—Cancer. 4. Language and medicine. 5. Justman, Stewart—Health. I. Title.

RC262 .J876 2003
362.1'96994—dc21   2002035106

To My Wife and Children

CONTENTS

Indeed there is but little difference between wisdom and medicine, and between all that is sought in wisdom and all that exists in medicine: contempt of money, honesty and modesty, simplicity in dress, respect, sound judgment, the spirit of decision, neatness, thoughtfulness, the knowledge of all that is necessary for life, hate of vice, the negation of superstitious fear of the gods, divine excellence.

—Hippocrates

PREFACE: CANCER AND CANT

IN WORLD WAR I, slaughter beyond precedent and previous imagining took place on a continent that believed itself the summit of civilization. But language did not necessarily keep up with reality. In England the approved way of describing the Great War was as a kind of Arthurian venture, a beautiful sacrifice, as though the event itself were part of a medieval revival. An entire vocabulary of anachronisms was employed. According to the "system of high diction" in force during the war, horses were steeds, actions deeds, soldiers warriors, sleep slumber, the sky the heavens, the front the field, corpses dust. This romantic lexicon was not invented on the spot. During the Victorian decades, advocates of heroic striving had urged upon a modern nation the values of knights-at-arms. Let us unite "in the true spirit of chivalry," wrote an editor of Thomas Malory. "We must remember that our nineteenth-century world is yet far from cleared of the monstrous powers of evil, which still oppress and devour the weak." Thus was an industrial society recalled to the virtues of Arthur. More general allusions to the romance tradition pervaded Victorian discourse. Whether as a result of these, the influence of Tennyson, or the chivalric mood and tenor of high Victorian culture generally, a language more suitable to a horse-riding aristocracy than a modern army carried into World War I, the cataclysm that marked the real end of the Victorian age.

Some of the language surrounding cancer seems to me just as out of keeping as this Arthurian depiction of modern warfare. Indeed, cancer itself is envisioned as warfare, with patients battling the disease and honored with the rhetoric of heroism. Cancer has its own high diction. Those who die of breast cancer "are said to have 'lost their battle' and may be memorialized by photographs carried at races for the cure—our lost, brave sisters, our fallen soldiers." The races themselves—staged as fundraisers—vaguely recall the funeral games of the *Iliad*. For their part, cancer patients who live are sometimes said to have conquered the disease but are more commonly termed survivors, like those who somehow emerge with their lives from a scene of disaster. "And I only am escaped alone to tell thee." A self-identified survivor of prostate cancer, and member of Congress, likens the moment he was told he had cancer to being shot down over North Vietnam. From this comparison one would never guess that many prostate cancers (and the same is true of breast cancers) come to nothing. The survivors weren't necessarily about to die in the first place. At times, it seems, cancer fires blanks. If there is heroism in cancer, so too is there something of the anti-heroic and the humiliating.

Any cancer patient would be glad to have the disease in remission, but according to some of the healers who make their voices heard in the literature, remission alone isn't enough. Unless the patient's mind is made healthy, "whether the tumor shrinks or even goes into complete remission, genuine healing will not have occurred." The better to know their own minds and "make room for new feelings," patients are urged to keep a journal. In the strange world of writing to, for, and of the self, memory of the wider scope of the written word seems to fall away. For all of its echoes of the heroic, cancer language itself introduces usages that seem completely new to human experience, at times giving the impression that the records of the past have been rubbed out and written over, the dream of a Year One realized. It is said, for example, that the prostate cancer patient needs to go through the stages of grieving. In the literature of the past people do not grieve for themselves. Only the dead can be grieved, that is, mourned. Not even Job grieves for himself. He curses, rages in misery, accuses, maintains his innocence, wishes for death, but he does not grieve as if for his own death. In the last book of the *Iliad* Priam, the king of Troy, is portrayed in grief for his unburied son Hector.

> The sons sitting around their father inside the courtyard
> made their clothes sodden with their tears, and among them
>   the old man
> sat veiled, beaten into his mantle. Dung lay thick on the head
>   and neck of the aged man, for he had been rolling
> in it, he had gathered and smeared it on with his hands.

That is grief. According to the counselors, the last step of a properly conducted grieving process is putting the past behind you. While that may or may not be, verbal inventions like "grieving for yourself" certainly put the usages of the past behind them.

Alienated from the past and in search of a source of strength in the face of a terrifying disease, some cancer patients look to the promises of mysticism and depth psychology. When first diagnosed with the disease himself, Michael Milken, the notorious financier and the leading advocate and private funder of prostate cancer research in the United States, studied meditation under Deepak Chopra. In Chopra's *Perfect Health: The Complete Mind Body Guide* (sic), readers are instructed to envision their body not

> as a collection of cells, tissues, and organs . . . [but] as a silent flow of intelligence, a constant bubbling up of impulses that create, control, and become your physical body. The secret of life at this level is that *anything in your body* can be changed with the flick of an intention.

How many cancer patients have been led to hope their disease could be cleared "with the flick of an intention"? But whatever their medical value, cures like those offered by Deepak Chopra do not cure the rootlessness that creates the audience for such things in the first place. Only those estranged from tradition would think of a tradition not as something you belong to but something you make use of, like a financier practicing meditation for his health.

In common with many others—for even the world of cancer is swept by trends and fashions—Michael Milken thinks stress may have had something to do with his disease. Many suspect stress of playing a part in cancer, many don't; but the cancer literature in any case has nothing good to say about stress. The theory that the good life is a life of ease, without tension and trial, would have been denied by Milton with all his strength.

> I cannot praise a fugitive and cloistered virtue, unexercised and unbreathed, that never sallies out and sees her adversary, but slinks out of the race where that immortal garland is to be run for, not without dust and heat.

That Milton does not have in mind the released tension of physical contests, like the games held in honor of Patroclus in the *Iliad*, simply confirms the importance he attaches to stress. For that matter, Odysseus himself, the original survivor, rejected the offer of a life of eternal ease on Calypso's island. He could have lived forever, stress-free, and elected not to. Certainly some have defended the contemplative life, but not, I imagine, because of the health benefits of contemplation. Cancer patients who actually followed the advice of the day regarding stress, meditation, diet, exercise, journal-writing, and support groups would be so obsessed with disease that the pursuit of health would become their sickness.

At the far left end of the cancer literature you encounter neologisms, one after another, whose only purpose seems to be to proclaim a break with common or traditional usage. Instead of writing about the body an author "writes the body." Direct action, direct object. A body that is some kind of cultural artifact, like a page of writing, is a verbal invention in its own right. Even in the mainstream literature it seems to go without saying that tradition is a spell to be broken. Cancer language sometimes judges the past as a whole—prostate or breast cancer "awareness" implying, for example, that the age of ignorance is at an end, or ought to be, and that the mystery and silence traditionally surrounding these diseases are pernicious in themselves. While none would deny the advances of medical knowledge and treatment, the prostate or breast cancer patient comes to learn that ignorance is by no means behind us, and that the liberating power of "awareness" has been overstated. The same critical spirit that guides medicine might also lead us to question the master-myth of our own culture's liberation from the errors of the past (and especially, perhaps, the Victorian past). It is because the past represents to me more than a record of ignorance and error that I refer to works of literature and art in the coming pages.

In a guide to living with cancer we are introduced to one

"Thomas O., a professor of English literature," diagnosed with prostate cancer at age sixty-two. In marked contrast to the workings of literature itself, but characteristically for this genre, we get to know almost nothing about Thomas O.—is he married? does he have children? does he have passions? just who is he?—but are nonetheless let into his most private thoughts. To his friends he confides,

> I've read and written about some of the greatest authors in the English language. I always imagined that I understood what they were saying when they described the tragedies of human existence. Now they seem to be hollow and meaningless. Their problems belonged to them. I have my own.

Perhaps this professor's interests restricted him to English writings, but would anyone say of Tolstoy's *Death of Ivan Ilych* that it was hollow and meaningless? As a teacher of literature myself, I can only state that throughout my own illness the memory of literature never left me, and when I read in some advice manual about, say, grief or choice, I could not but envision characters grieving and choosing. To devalue the past is to impoverish the present, and so it is, perhaps, that threadbare phrases and bankrupt consolations fill the cancer literature as if they were not themselves null and void. The title attached to the story of Thomas O. is "Life Is Beautiful."

The same guide to cancer reminds the patient that

> by definition, heroes are uncommon. Most of us are quite ordinary. Nevertheless, in each of us is the potential for the heroic, expressed in our individual way.

Like a child with a workbook, the reader is encouraged to ask, "What kind of hero lies within me?" In *The Death of Ivan Ilych*, the tale of a man of no distinction who accidentally becomes a sort of tragic hero, it is as if Tolstoy brought the full force of his imagination to bear on the proposition that an ordinary person can rise to the heroic. The result, however, is a work of great and bitter irony, not of inspirational nostrums. Exactly for this reason, the story of Ivan Ilych is discussed at some length later in these pages.

Some decades ago the civil rights movement challenged the nation and heightened public awareness of oppression. Strangely, a similar rhetoric of liberation has come into use in the cancer world. Now it is cancer patients who challenge an unwritten law that the disease is to remain in the shadows and who, battling that disease in a kind of moral equivalent of war, also advance in some way the interests of humanity. Voices of both the breast and prostate cancer "communities" proclaim the importance of breaking a tradition of silence and of bringing the public to a new understanding; and they proclaim this over and over, like a Dickens character with a mechanical refrain. To my mind, at any rate, the adoption of the idiom of liberation in the cancer world results in a rhetoric stylized and unreal. How such rhetoric took root I don't know; but, repeating as it does themes already well into their second generation, it certainly has the attraction of familiarity. Perhaps the familiarity of liberation rhetoric serves to keep the overwhelming strangeness of cancer at bay somehow—a dike against the sea. Conventions of rhetoric, approved formulas of political argument, warm clichés of psychology—all have been deployed against this force that attacks "places where we breathe / And love and think of what cannot be true." In the case of this patient, fear flashed through the body, hope ebbed and surged, gratitude for acts of kindness found no speech, a new persuasion arose that the functions of the body could no longer be taken for granted and might disappear, like something both precious and treacherous, and these events took place as though the institutional rhetoric of cancer simply did not exist.

Like death itself, disease is a great equalizer, a leveler of distinctions. Both Michael Milken and the prosecutor who sent him to prison have had prostate cancer. A president of France suffered with prostate cancer in office. One of my physicians is herself a cancer patient. While men and women wrangle over equality, breast and prostate cancer in the United States pose equivalent numbers and equivalent dilemmas. Not only does cancer override differences like a tide washing over a fortress of sand, it subverts our pride, ignores our fashions, tests our certainties.

SEEDS OF MORTALITY

POLLS, STATISTICS, FORMS

IN A STUDY of deception published not long after the Watergate affair and the crisis of trust occasioned by it, Sissela Bok tells of a man in his forties who makes a routine visit to his doctor, not knowing that he has incurable cancer. The doctor, once he makes the discovery, must decide whether and how much to tell the patient. "Even if he does reveal the serious nature of the diagnosis, should he mention the possibility of chemotherapy and his reasons for not recommending it in this case? Or should he encourage every last effort to postpone death?"

In this case the doctor told half the truth, informing the patient of his condition but concealing the option of chemotherapy. To that extent he lied; but what offends Sissela Bok isn't just the lie but the freedom to lie or not, as he sees fit, in the first place. Unchecked power invites abuse. Sissela Bok would like to restrict the right to lie to certain narrowly defined, exceptional cases (the case of the unsuspecting forty-year-old not being one). In order for a medical lie to be defensible, moreover, its necessity must be established not just in the doctor's mind but to the satisfaction of other minds—other doctors, nurses, patients themselves. That is, the rationale for lying must be capable of being made public. As Kant says, a motive

> which I may not *declare openly* without thereby frustrating my own intention, or which must at all costs be *kept secret* if it is to succeed, or which I cannot *publicly acknowledge* without thereby arousing the resistance of everyone to my plans, can only have stirred up this necessary and general . . . opposition against me because it is itself unjust and thus constitutes a threat to everyone.

Just as the Kantian norm of Law lies a long way from the world of lawyers and lawsuits better known to us, so too what Kant terms the "transcendental principle of publicness" differs widely from publicity as we know it—commercials, public relations exercises, press releases, public awareness campaigns, the sea of simplifications in which we all swim. Publicity in the common sense of the word is something that can't be contemplated without some measure of irony, some feeling for the ridiculous, which Kant may have lacked but someone who gets seriously ill soon acquires.

As lucid, intelligent, and morally correct as it is, Sissela Bok's proposal to restrict the physician's right to lie must itself be taken with a grain of irony. In reply to the argument that patients don't want to hear bad news (for if they did, the doctor who conceals the truth would simply be complying with their wishes), Sissela Bok contends that as a matter of fact most patients *would* like to know the worst. "In most of the studies, over 80 percent of the persons asked indicated that they would want to be told." What does it mean for people to indicate they would want to be told of an incurable illness? To my mind this "would want" is simply too speculative, too imaginary, as though the truth could be reached through a game of pretend. Put to the healthy, the question "Would you like to know you have cancer?" is play-acting; put to the cancer patient, the question "Would you prefer not to know you have cancer?" practically answers itself, because not-knowing is no help and no option. One question is fanciful, the other derisive. Evidently this is a matter that just doesn't lend itself to opinion polls. Had I been asked the question in good health, certainly I would have said that I'd want to know the whole truth, if only because any other reply is too shameful. As it happened, when I was diagnosed with cancer, there were many things I didn't inquire about. Also, words like "cure" and "incurable" were not used. Reality didn't fit the grid. The reality of cancer also reduced all hypotheticals to an exercise in make-believe, like the question of what you would do if you came upon a burning building or a drowning man. It is said that conservatism, at its origin, distrusts "all that may smack of speculation or hypothesis." The conservative or just the skeptic in me questions such pipedream data as the fact that most people, on the evidence of a mark in a box, are willing to look death in the eye.

Experience humbles, instructs, transforms us. Before the fact I never would have imagined allowing a surgeon to learn on me; in the event, I did. If experience conformed to our preconceptions, the masters of literature might never have bothered with its portrayal at all. Until tested by experience, some of our capacities remain unproven and some, like courage, cannot fairly be said to exist at all. Projected courage is armchair courage. Courage exists in action and nowhere else, so that the only way to find out if someone has courage is to wait and see. To forecast or pretend to forecast acts of courage amounts to an attempt to rip the veil from the future. It is an act of impatience. And to ask people if they would want to be told of a mortal illness comes close to asking if they intend to show

courage—or, even more absurdly, if they would prefer being courageous to being cowardly.

To be sure, years ago when I first read Sissela Bok's study of
lies and liars, I thought about what it would be like to be diagnosed
with an incurable disease. But how is it possible to capture thought
itself in an opinion survey? How can something so private, shadowy,
and unformed be registered as a check mark? How can the silent
dialogue of reflection be transcribed into the public idiom of yes
and no? Like attaching my name to a plea for more funding for cancer research, such a poll standardizes the responses it records by
placing them into ready-made categories. My own mortality in particular is a matter too intimate for position-taking and too profound
to be figured statistically. None of this deterred Gallup. In 1979 a
Gallup Poll was conducted in which people were actually asked not
whether they have confidence in the economy, not whether they
split their ticket, but whether they would want to be told if they had
an incurable illness. Between 82 and 92 percent of adults, "depending on sex, race, education, age, income, and occupation," said yes.
The numbers mean little, but that such a question could be asked at
all is revealing, implying as it does a belief that the truth can be cap-
tured with the crudest instruments and that even the most private
topics lend themselves to public representation.

Besides, two can play at polling. Another poll reveals men with
some understanding of prostate cancer but greatly underestimating
their own chances of it, almost as though the same people who
"would want" to be informed of a fatal condition refused to recognize their liability to a condition potentially just that. Such polls
support the belief that men are living in a state of denial, of delib-
erate ignorance—a paradoxically fashionable belief that goes quite
contrary to the image of open-eyed fearlessness favored by Sissela

Bok. I can't shake the thought that both sorts of polls generate exactly the data they were intended to. It is the practice of asking leading questions in a show of investigation that produces such knots. Although polls are said to show that a percentage of the respondents think this or think that, they misrepresent what it is to think in the first place.

In *The Brothers Karamazov* Dostoevsky tells of a painting entitled "Contemplation."

> There is a forest in winter, and on a roadway through the forest, in absolute solitude, stands a peasant in a torn kaftan and bark shoes. He stands, as it were, lost in thought. Yet he is not thinking; he is "contemplating." If anyone touched him he would start and look at one as though awakening and bewildered. It's true he would come to himself immediately; but if he were asked what he had been thinking about, he would remember nothing. Yet probably he has hidden within himself, the impression which had dominated him during the period of contemplation.

Or as Iris Murdoch says less darkly, "The task of attention goes on all the time and at apparently empty and everyday moments we are 'looking,' making those little peering efforts of imagination which have such important cumulative results." If someone hands me a form asking what I think about my mortality, that is one thing. The actual process of thinking takes place at another level, imperceptible at times even to me, quiet and gradual but potentially decisive like the accumulation of snow or the process of erosion. The communion of the mind with itself is too subtle for the categories and instruments of the opinion survey. And the notion that cancer has anything to do with public opinion seems to me that much more far-fetched because the disease itself can be so secretive. Symptom-less, invisible to the world but potentially lethal, cancer is the all but unspeakable secret I bore and perhaps still bear in my body—the word behind the word, the thought behind the thought, the hum beneath the other noises. Inside the body of the unsuspecting forty-year-old, cancer had a life of its own. With me, cancer almost has thoughts of its own. In keeping my condition from others I became a black parody of a pregnant woman who keeps to herself the secret of her joy. Polls, pink ribbons, public service announcements, even the pro and con of medical opinion on the op-ed pages came as if from another world.

To question the claim that patients want to know the worst because surveys indicate that they do (as if patients themselves were exempt from lying) isn't to say that doctors should go ahead and de-ceive their patients. Hippocrates is right: doctors ought to be both honest and modest. They can't be either if they reserve the right to lie whenever they deem it in the patient's interest to be deceived. But no rules and no procedures exist that will make people honest or modest. As it happens, the doctor who told me of my condition is both of these things to a wonderful degree. Dr. Green speaks with a bit of a drawl and has a boyish face lit up from within by a sort of subtle Chaucerian smile. As with Chaucer, a lot of his comments are pitched between the serious and the comic—fittingly, because prostate cancer entails so much not only of the ominous but the ridiculous. With his unassuming skill and his way of never lecturing or shaming or pretending to be above the condition he treats, Dr. Green reminds you in his own person of the bond that once existed between humanism and medicine. Without the least evasion or re-luctance, but also without the least doubt of his own skill, he con-fessed that he was still learning the surgical procedure that would be

performed on me and so would have to be supervised in the operating room. Yet the same man made a mockery of disclosure in the
act of securing my informed consent. Reading a legal form listing
the risks I was agreeing to was less like having facts illuminated than
like having a light directed into my own eyes. Such shows of respect
for informed consent are better than the deception of an unsuspecting patient—but not that much better.

SISSELA BOK writes of doctors who lie at their own discretion and
with complete impunity. Whether or not this is a just image of the
medical profession at some time in the past, by now the author's plea
for honesty has lost much of its point. If my case is in any way typ-
ical, patients today are going to be informed of all the probabilities
(with numbers assigned)—not because the doctors have become
Kantians but simply because they are covering themselves legally.
While their disclosure forms serve to bewilder and defeat the
signer—that is, to frustrate the ends of disclosure itself—they suc-
ceed in protecting the physician or the hospital against legal action.
In this age of the lawsuit you can't get a flu shot without immu-
nizing the clinic. The age is so litigious that medical advocates of
screening for prostate cancer remind their opponents within the
profession of the lawsuits filed and won against their kind. Doctors
threaten doctors with lawyers. "The debate has moved from the
doctor's office into the courthouse." Even a cancer guide advising
patients to get in touch with their subconscious and talk with their
disease has the sense to post a legal disclaimer: "This book is meant
to educate and should not be used as an alternative for professional
medical care [etc.]." Professional care brings its own legalities. A
consent form, for example, is legal armor, and like a pharmaceutical

ad with tracts of unreadably small print, it turns the very act of disclosure into a method of disinformation.

The consent form I was given to sign by Dr. Green the day before surgery reads in part:

PERMISSION FOR SURGICAL CARE

VERIFICATION OF INFORMED CONSENT

I hereby authorize and direct William J. Green, MD, with associates or assistants of his choice, to perform the following operation:

TRANSPERINEAL BRACHYTHERAPY AND CYSTOSCOPY

I further authorize the doctor(s) to do any other procedure that their judgment may dictate to be necessary or advisable should unforeseen circumstances arise during the operation. The details of the operation or procedure have been explained to me in terms that I could understand. Alternative methods of treatment, if any, have been explained to me, as have benefits and disadvantages of each. We have also discussed the risks, if any, of not having the operation or procedure. I am advised that though good results are expected, complications cannot be anticipated and that therefore there can be no guarantee, either expressed or implied, as to the results of the surgery or cure. The doctor has answered all my questions.

The doctor has explained to me the most likely complications or problems that might occur in this operation and during the healing period, and I understand them. Those risks include: **Bleeding requiring transfusion of my blood or of Blood bank blood, risks of anesthesia, hematoma, infection, death, blood clots in the legs with possible blood clot to the lungs (pulmonary embolus), graft, urinary leakage, renal failure, urinary re-**

tention, frequency or urgency of urination, slowed stream, impotence, incontinence, rectal irritation or fistula, failure of the procedure to correct the initiating problem and other risks associated with major surgery. [Etc.]

Hamlet was right, then. There *is* something after death.

I fail to see that this document is really that much more informative than a traditional lie. Looking at it is like staring into a blizzard. With such a thing before you, there is nothing to do but ignore it and sign. Owing to the nature of the surgery itself, I had to sign. Brachytherapy refers to the implantation of radioactive pellets, or "seeds," and when the order for these had been placed some weeks before, I signed another form promising payment in full even if, for some reason, I were to cancel the surgery. In the spirit of full disclosure, the radiation oncologist advised that in signing I would be liable for $7,000. Had I not signed the consent form in Dr. Green's office, I would have been left with untreated cancer plus a mighty bill for titanium seeds that had been calibrated for my case and no other.

A document telling me that good results are looked for but I might die doesn't inform me; but it was never really designed to inform. It was designed for the legal security of the physician. Being a legal instrument, the consent form has spaces not only for my signature but a witness's. It records my consent but also the "verification" of that consent, as if a door were being double-locked. "Authorize and direct," or for that matter "operation or procedure," seems a legal doublet like "cease and desist." And who but a lawyer would have written "there can be no guarantee, either expressed or implied"? (Similarly, it must have been for purely legal purposes that I had to certify that the doctor used simple words and answered all questions.) No patient would sign such a contract who didn't simply trust the physician, as unscientific as the traditional sentiment of trust may be.

In the past some doctors lied about cancer in the belief that it was better for the patient not to know. Today a doctor who thought it better for a patient's peace of mind not to know about prostate cancer wouldn't screen for it in the first place—a policy actually recommended by the Centers for Disease Control on the grounds that so little is reliably known about this inscrutable disease as well as its treatment. The doctor who doesn't look for prostate cancer can achieve the results of lying without ever uttering an untrue word. These days not many doctors would be foolhardy enough to lie to their patients with the frankness, as it were, of former times. My own physicians, who looked to what could be done instead of what couldn't be known, did not prevaricate. But just as "It really is of importance, not only what men do, but also what manner of men they are that do it," as John Stuart Mill wrote, so do the reasons for an act—in this case the act of disclosure—really matter. When patients are warned of risks not because they are owed this information as human beings but because the physician wants to be armed against the risks of legal action, the act of disclosure is perverted into a legal maneuver. It is ironic that Sissela Bok overlooked this possibility, as one of the works prominently cited by her—a classic of world literature—exposes doctors and lawyers as doubles under the skin.

PRECEDING Sissela Bok's essay on "Lies to the Sick and Dying" is an epigraph from Tolstoy's *The Death of Ivan Ilych*:

This deception tortured him—their not wishing to admit what they all knew and what he knew, but wanting to lie to him concerning his terrible condition, and wishing and forcing him to participate in that lie. Those lies—lies enacted over him on the eve of his death and destined to degrade this awful, solemn act to the level of their visitings, their curtains, their sturgeon for dinner—were a terrible agony for Ivan Ilych.

In *The Death of Ivan Ilych* we read of a successful careerist, petty, imitative, shallow, outstanding in nothing, who in the course of a mortal illness slowly awakens to the horror of his own misspent life. At the height of his good fortune Ivan Ilych holds the position of a judge. As such he views those who come before him as cases, that is, not as persons but problems or illustrations. Only when he himself becomes a case—a medical case—in consequence of a slip on a stepladder, does the ordeal of his awakening begin. So it is that *The Death of Ivan Ilych* turns upon the equivalence of the physician and the lawyer as figures of pride and pretension. About this correspondence Tolstoy is perfectly explicit:

> He went [to the doctor]. Everything took place as he had expected and as it always does. There was the usual waiting and the important air assumed by the doctor, with which he was so familiar (resembling that which he himself assumed in court), and the sounding and listening, and the questions which called for answers that were foregone conclusions and were evidently unnecessary, and the look of importance which implied that "if only you put yourself in our hands we will arrange everything—we know indubitably how it has to be done, always the same for everybody." It was all just as it was

in the law courts. The doctor put on just the same air towards him as he himself put on towards an accused person.

Though written in the third person, this passage reflects in some degree Ivan Ilych's own perceptions. In the doctor's air of professional detachment and competent authority Ivan Ilych sees his own manner, even as he senses that this man is of no possible use to him. The experience is repeated with other doctors, all of them reflecting back his own demeanor in court, none of them able to treat or even understand his disease, or much reduce his pain. It is as though Ivan Ilych peered into a clouded mirror, discerning in these others what he cannot yet recognize in himself—fraudulence. Ivan Ilych perceives that these men are impostors, and even perceives that he is like them, but not until the end does he bow to the inescapable conclusion that he too has been an impostor. Only after long agony does the force of the argument "He is false; I am just like him; therefore I too am false" come home to Ivan Ilych.

Luckily or unluckily, Ivan Ilych undergoes his ordeal without anyone at his side to assure him that "denial, anger, fear, shock, disbelief, regret, confusion, helplessness, panic, worry, depression, grief" are "perfectly understandable and normal" reactions to cancer. Ivan Ilych experiences most of these things without having them labeled and professionally validated. By analogy with the physician challenged to heal himself, a judge undergoes a trial. In *The Kreutzer Sonata*, written in the same decade, Tolstoy sets up another resemblance between the two professions. Of doctors the tale's principal narrator says,

> They have ruined my life as they have ruined and are ruining the lives of thousands and hundreds of thousands of human beings, and I cannot help connecting the effect with the cause.

I understand that they want to earn money like lawyers and others, and I would willingly give them half my income, and all who realize what they are doing would willingly give them half their possessions, if only they would not interfere with our family life and would never come near us.

Whatever Tolstoy's private obsession with doctors and lawyers, the fact is that satire itself has paired the two professions at least since Chaucer's portrayal of the Physician and the Sergeant of Law as men of wealth who talk up their own learning. In the eyes of satire, it seems, the physician and the lawyer are twins, both swollen with the pride of false knowledge, both given to lying, both plagues to those unlucky enough to find themselves in their power. In the land of the horses, says Gulliver, "was neither physician to destroy my body, nor lawyer to ruin my fortune." But what pertinence do these fine caricatures have today, when doctors do much good, in contrast to the no good at all they do Ivan Ilych? Many in our culture seem to believe that those who walked the earth before us walked in darkness; that the past is one long spell of ignorance and repression, from which we ourselves have been delivered. Some might say the portrayal of doctors as greedy charlatans, tormentors of body and soul, belongs to a bygone age and is itself a product of backwardness.

Ivan Ilych's doctors differ among themselves and can't seem to decide whether the trouble is his kidney or his appendix. Disagreements over prostate cancer go so deep that they bring to mind descriptions of the novel as that literary form where everything is contested. As a layman I had no idea medical science housed differences of opinion this fundamental. Only belatedly did I learn that in the urological world there are those who believe in screening for and treating prostate cancer and those who seriously question the point of screening and even treatment. The Centers for Disease Control discourage early screening, the American Cancer Society urges it, and the American Urological Association divides the baby by stating that early detection has both "advantages and disadvantages" and "may be important." Some years ago, by a twist of circumstance, I found myself with two urologists, a doubter and a doer. The former judged the latter unprofessional. A friend who saw his dissertation director die of prostate cancer goes to a doctor who doesn't bother with the blood test for the disease (the prostate-specific antigen, or PSA). In Britain, it seems, they do not routinely do the PSA either. The prostate cancer patient hears that this is a disease men die "with and not of." He also hears that advanced prostate cancer is not pretty and that more than thirty thousand die of the disease each year in the United States. Well before meeting Dr. Green and certainly before looking into the issue or even knowing there was an issue, I had already made a choice in effect between the do-nothing and the do-something approaches to prostate cancer. By having blood tests and biopsies, I cast my lot with activism. For his part, Dr. Green never mentioned the other faction's doubts regarding the aggressive treatment of prostate cancer, either because of my age or possibly because he considered such doubts moot as I had already waived the option of inaction by seeking his services in the first place. It is ironic, anyway, that in the case of this patient informed consent originated in ignorance.

When I began getting tested for prostate cancer, I had never heard of the arguments against testing—the publicity being one-sided—and by the time I was diagnosed it was too late to go back and pretend there was no point in looking for the disease. I had made my decision without ever being aware of making it. In this matter of prostate cancer, something can be said for not seeking after knowledge, not getting screened at all. What became clear to me is that I had already decided otherwise and must now accept the results for better or worse. "There is and can be no *beginning* to any event, for one event always flows uninterruptedly from another," says Tolstoy in *War and Peace*. Just so, my choice was made before I can remember making one, and revealed itself only in retrospect. (In *The Death of Ivan Ilych* itself, only belatedly do the hero and the reader recognize his mishap on the stepladder as the onset of his decline. In real time the event passes almost unnoticed.) Elsewhere Tolstoy speaks of the chess player who imagines a game won or lost on the strength of some single move, rather than an accumulation of small moves. With little or no thinking I had made some early moves that set the course of the game.

In accordance with Tolstoy's denial of absolute beginnings, we are probably to take Ivan Ilych's accident on the stepladder as the last straw—the final, critical event in a series of events—not the sole cause of his fatal illness. The illness itself is simply beyond the competence of medicine. Other than opium, the doctors have no treatment for Ivan Ilych, and so one can't really say their treatment is worse than the disease; but on the other hand the tale intimates that if Ivan Ilych hadn't been so much like them he might not have fallen ill to begin with. Symbolically speaking, the physicians *are* his disease. While Tolstoy certainly believes the doctors' methods useless (like the waters prescribed for Kitty in *Anna Karenina*), something in him agrees with Gulliver that medicine is worse than useless—it is ruinous. Ironically, though, medicine itself long ago recognized that some cancers are better left untreated. In this honorable tradition of medical conservatism going back to Hippocrates and Galen stand the critics of the overtreatment of prostate cancer. In their view, much of the treatment of the disease is of uncertain value and some positively destructive. They are right. We have not outgrown Tolstoy, it seems. But perhaps the critics of medical overzealousness and the counselors of inaction would also do well to reflect on the tale of Ivan Ilych. Their arguments rest on statistics and the lack of them; but if cancer showed up in their body, would they follow their own arguments and do nothing about it? Or would they, like Ivan Ilych, change their thinking when the implications of their position came home to them and they became patients themselves?

Even if medicine spoke with one voice about prostate cancer, the satiric portrayal of folly, pretension, deceit, and greed would retain its point as long as these things remain with us. The notion that satiric categories and evaluations not only belong to the past but impede human progress—in my view this is a utopian delusion that only satire itself could do justice to.

At the end of his consultation with "a celebrated doctor," Ivan Ilych places the doctor's fee on the table. Before even meeting my radiation oncologist, Dr. Marion, who would be doing the surgery with Dr. Green, I was put on notice that fees would be high and would not conform to Blue Cross guidelines. Still in the waiting room, I was handed a sheet entitled HOW DO WE SET OUR FEES? which began:

> Today, you are seeing a radiation oncologist at the Cancer Center. Our physicians have specialty training in radiation oncology, and their fees reflect this expertise.

This seemed ominous. The form is in fact a socially conscious expression of greed—the policy statement of people not at ease with the idea of gouging patients ("There is no question cancer treatments can be very expensive"), but determined all the same to make a great deal of money. Here was a disclosure form that served a warning. One of Dr. Marion's technicians had a satiric streak of his own. In order to complete a difficult bit of imaging that had to be done in planning the surgery, this craftsman used rubber bands. "But these are no ordinary rubber bands," he said. "These are $750 rubber bands."

WITH PHYSICIANS so mindful of the risks of lawsuits, Sissela Bok's argument against a medical right to lie has become largely moot. But in point of fact it was already being overtaken by events in 1979 when her book first appeared. Asking people if they would want to be told they were dying is a charade—because they are not dying; but asking doctors whether in fact they lie to patients has some value. In surveys of physicians conducted over the 1970s, the heavy majorities that once existed in favor of a right to lie disappeared. Indeed, by the year *Lying: Moral Choice in Public and Private Life* was published, the reversal of opinion was "virtually complete." Heavy majorities now opposed discretionary lying. If the surveys are to be believed (and in fact even if they are not), by the time Sissela Bok recorded the case of the patient who was told half the truth, medical opinion had already turned definitely toward a policy of disclosure. Is this because the medical profession suddenly felt the force of excellent arguments? Doubtful. Medical opinion shifted with the times. Much like those social critics who raise a cry against patriarchy at a time when many families contain no father, or who redouble their attacks on racism at a time when racism itself has been officially discredited, Sissela Bok devastates the arguments of her opponents at a moment when they themselves—their number dwindling—are rapidly losing confidence in their position. They are doing so because the "credibility gap" has become a public topic, because paternalism itself has lost its credibility—in brief, because opinion in general has turned against those who abuse trust by lying. Interestingly, though, in *The Death of Ivan Ilych* the ability to turn with the times and adopt properly liberal opinions is portrayed not as the sign of an enlightened mind but as one more evidence of shallowness and opportunism. An opening presented itself to the young Ivan Ilych when "the new and reformed judicial institutions were introduced, and new men were needed. Ivan Ilych became such a new man." The physicians who overthrew traditional medical views on lying were not necessarily more thoughtful or compassionate than those who came before them. They too were new men. Those who may have lied on their survey forms simply in order to register the correct opinions were much like Ivan Ilych, himself correct in all things. But if the views of physicians are subject to trends of opinion, so too are those of patients.

"In most of the studies, over 80 percent of the persons asked indicated that they would want to be told." It is, again, ironic that public opinion should be cited as authoritative in an essay that has at its head a passage from *The Death of Ivan Ilych,* for public opinion was the ruin of Ivan Ilych. "I was going up in public opinion, but to the same extent life was ebbing away from me. And now it's all over and there's only death." (Nor is there anything incidental or shallow-rooted about Tolstoy's hostility to public opinion in *The Death of Ivan Ilych.* A strong strain of Rousseau runs through the novella from beginning to end, and Rousseau's *Émile* is preserved from any kind of dependence on opinion. Tolstoy thought *Émile* the best treatise on education in existence.) Had some survey asked whether I would want to be told of my impending death, I would know without a moment's doubt that the enlightened answer to this question—the correct answer, the only reportable answer—is yes, and would produce that answer in the same spirit of doing the proper thing that destroys Ivan Ilych, as Tolstoy makes painfully clear. A statement like "Studies show that people want to be informed they are dying" is one Tolstoy himself would satirize ruthlessly, as he satirizes newspapers in *The Death of Ivan Ilych* and history books in *War and Peace*. Despising pretenders, Tolstoy would not think much of surveys that ask people to pretend they are dying.

The passage from *The Death of Ivan Ilych* cited by Sissela Bok depicts a hero surrounded by people who refuse to acknowledge that he is dying and torment him with their lies. He craves the truth. By this time, though, Ivan Ilych has been dying for three months. In the earlier stages of his decline it was different. "In the depth of his heart he knew he was dying, but not only was he unaccustomed to the thought, he simply did not and could not grasp it." In fact, even after his mind rebels against the lies encircling him, Ivan Ilych still cannot reconcile himself to the thought of death. He reaches for false hope again and again. Looking back to the onset of his illness as he approaches its end, Tolstoy writes: "From the very beginning of his illness, ever since he had first been to see the doctor, Ivan Ilych's life had been divided between two contrary and alternating moods, either despair and the expectation of this uncomprehended and terrible death, or hope. . . ." This portrayal of a man pulled two ways, as on a rack, seems to me more convincing and even more truthful than the survey data cited in "Lies to the Sick and Dying." Human beings are not transparent. Our core—the depth of our hearts—does not disclose itself to opinion surveys. "In most of the studies, over 80% of the persons asked indicated that they would want to know." Let this exemplify the distortion and the unreality that set in when the most private crises of our experience, such as sickness, supply matter for public debate. Just as honesty is transformed into something like its own opposite on a standard disclosure form, so our thoughts about death can't be fitted into the standard categories of an opinion survey without a loss of truth.

REFLECTING ON the nature of the good, Iris Murdoch faults the philosophers' reduction of moral choice to an empty act, and the corresponding impoverishment of the moral lexicon. Instead of saying simply "This is right" or "I choose this," we ought to say, "'This is A B C D' (normative-descriptive words), and action will follow naturally." That is, instead of investing all in a single absolute term like "choose" or "right," it would make sense to employ more varied and informative, more novelistic language. According to Sissela Bok, "Honesty from health professionals matters more to patients than almost everything else that they experience when ill." But this is practically to crown honesty king—to raise it into the single supreme term governing moral practice. Sincerity has its own traps. Rousseau, starting with a belief in his own sincerity, ends in paranoid delusion. A breast cancer organization proclaims in its statement of principles, "We are not afraid to examine all sides of all issues" and "We tell the truth about what we discover," as though its implied indictment of others as liars and cowards and its grievance against "the American medical establishment" were somehow less questionable than the ordinary politics of accusation. Iris Murdoch herself calls attention to the overvaluation of sincerity in modern philosophy. Honesty matters in a doctor; so do knowledge, skill, attentiveness, consideration, a sense of humor, humanity, humility. Nor would I care to list these attributes in order of importance. Honesty to the patient is just part of fidelity to the practice of medicine.

THE FAITHFUL PLOWMAN

AT THE AGE of fifty-three, a few days after a third biopsy in two years, I was diagnosed with that disease of old men, prostate cancer. Though it didn't sound like much cancer—"one millimeter"—in the next breath Dr. Green advised removal of the prostate altogether. (Later I learned there has been a great increase in radical prostatectomies, by some accounts a tripling, in recent years. When critics argue that the treatment is out of proportion to the disease, it is facts like these they have in mind.) Stunned as well as bewildered, I scheduled a conference the following week and hung up the phone. Over the next few days I pondered the possibilities, knowing the high incidence of dismal side effects following this operation and hoping for some third way in between no treatment at all (which one like Dr. Green will advise only if he thinks you will die of something else in the meantime) and surgery that would get rid of the cancer, probably, but could also do away with much else. I thought of the trapped beaver sacrificing his leg to save his life. When my wife and I met with Dr. Green to get our bearings and possibly settle on a course of treatment, it was September 12, 2001.

In the conference, Dr. Green first explained that the tumor had been upgraded on the scale of malignancy, then calculated my probabilities on the basis of this rating and a blood test. (The blood test put me in the worst category, but, he noted, just barely the worst. That was like him.) Finally he raised the option of implanting radioactive "seeds"—and all of this with patience, clarity, and gentleness. Unlike the doctor in *War and Peace* who "considered it his duty as a doctor to pose as a man whose every moment was of value to suffering humanity," Dr. Green just quietly did his work. A world had come to an end the day before, or at least an event so terrible had taken place that it made life before that date seem like the slumber of innocence, and Dr. Green went on with his duties as if nothing had happened. To me "business as usual" once signified a vicious rut, a kind of brute indifference, a willed blindness to reality—the daily operations of a town next to a concentration camp. Now it seemed more like fidelity to your calling. Thinking over this meeting, my mind went back to a beautiful and haunting visual parable of business as usual, Peter Brueghel's *Landscape with the Fall of Icarus*, painted around 1558.

The painting shows, in the foreground, a plowman following his ox, while off to the right, barely visible to us and outside the plowman's field of vision and consciousness, a single white leg plunges into the sea. Near a shepherd—also with his back turned to the disappearing leg—cluster a flock of fine sheep. A galleon sails by, but away from the leg, not toward it. A boy falls from the sky—an event that rips the fabric of reality, an event that could never have been imagined before it occurred—and nothing changes. The work of the world goes on.

Some no doubt will read *Landscape with the Fall of Icarus* as a comment on man's indifference to man. The way the world remains unchanged by the agony of the plunging figure will remind them

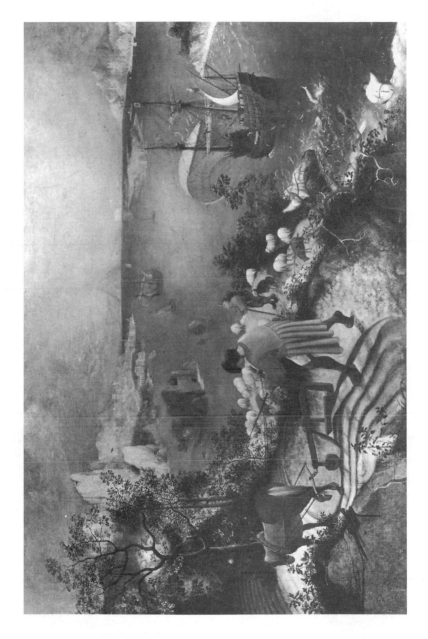

of the infamous New Yorkers of some decades ago who shut out the screams of their neighbor as she was knifed to death. For these viewers, the sight or the fact of human suffering is a siren that takes precedence over all else. On this showing, the painting depicts an emergency to which no one responds. But I wonder if such an interpretation of *Landscape with the Fall of Icarus* would ever suggest itself to a mind not already bound to a set of ideas about insensitivity to the sufferings of others. To construe the painting as a study of human callousness—in effect, an indictment of the plowman who attends to his own work—is not so much to read it as to impose on it beliefs that were already fully formed in the viewer's mind before the viewer ever laid eyes on it, beliefs that belong to an age well after the painter's own. Such a moralizing interpretation finds almost no support in the painting itself, for the plowman does not ignore suffering. To ignore is to pay no attention, to disregard, and the plowman is depicted not as disregarding the falling boy but as being simply unaware of him. The boy falls behind his back. Nor in any case can something be done about a boy plunging from the sky into the sea. He cannot be saved. This is not a pictorial sermon about a bad Samaritan.

To those enthralled by "the revelatory power of the extraordinary"—those who imagine that the truth "becomes manifest only in . . . extreme moments which 'ordinary life' covers over"—Brueghel's painting of a plowman who misses a revelation completely must be either an ironic proof of their thesis or an embarrassment. One reason some might take a prejudicial view of the plowman, in spite of the evidence of the painting itself, is the low value placed by the enlightened mind on repetitive labor and customary patterns. Among the images of stagnation used by John Stuart Mill in his essay *On Liberty* to depict the disgrace of blind habit is "the mill-horse round." Brueghel's plowman is like that horse, going round and round his land (to the left of the painting the furrows bend like the turn of a track) and although not wearing blinders, fixing his vision just ahead of his own feet as if he were. He bears a kind of humorous likeness to the plodding ox whose rump he follows. By now, though, the stultifying effect of habit and the invigorating effect of disruption have themselves become received ideas of the kind Mill complained of. Considering the example of Dr. Green, who carried out his daily routine with fidelity and precision at a moment when normalcy itself seemed shattered, I rethought my last remaining prejudices against the plowman.

"Business as usual" once suggested a vicious rut. But there does not seem to be anything vicious about the plowman, while the ruts, the grooves, he makes in the earth rhyme visually with the lovely folds of his own gown, as though both were expressions of human skill. "Business as usual" meant a willed blindness. But the plowman does not turn away from the falling figure; again, the figure falls behind his back, just as the sun that melted the boy's wings throws his shadow from behind. The plowman therefore shows no brute indifference, either. That he seems to be at one with the brute he is hitched to (his gown falling like the beast's tail) only means that he belongs to a harmonious order—and that this order survives undisturbed, in spite of any impression that the order of things is shattered by the unnatural event of a boy falling from the sky.

In the novels of Jane Austen, the great issues of the Napoleonic era, issues of war and peace, recede from view. The novels relegate to the remote background the events that occupy the center stage of history. Of Wickham and Lydia we learn at the end of *Pride and Prejudice* that "their manner of living, even when the restoration of peace dismissed them to a home, was unsettled in the extreme." You can read an Austen novel without remembering a passing reference to the slave trade. Like Brueghel, Jane Austen is interested in the very nature of notice. It is the cynical Mary Crawford who says in *Mansfield Park*, "I must look down upon anything contented with obscurity when it might rise to distinction." She says this in the presence of Fanny Price, the human image of the unnoticed. In *Landscape with the Fall of Icarus*, obscurity takes the form of an anonymous plowman, the ascent to distinction that of a boy who rose too high. Here one doing nothing out of the ordinary holds our eye while the spectacular event of a boy falling into the sea is so completely displaced into the background that it barely leaves a visual trace. Also set in the Napoleonic era, Tolstoy's *War and Peace* follows the principle that "the most important factors are the most ordinary occurrences," not the ones that receive the attention of historians or the acclaim of humanity. Ivan Ilych dies as a result of a mishap so ordinary it goes practically unnoticed. Gerasim, an important character in *The Death of Ivan Ilych*, escapes our eye at first, camouflaged almost to the point of invisibility. In fact, to Tolstoy's mind "what is noticed *cannot* be important." (Surely, therefore, Tolstoy would say that if you want to find the truth of people's attitude toward death, do not bother looking in newspapers or Gallup polls, things that exist solely to be noticed.) Maybe Peter Brueghel had a similar sense of where importance lies.

According to a folk tradition that extended into Brueghel's age, death is merely "an inevitable aspect of life itself, beyond which life triumphed and continued again." Death therefore is to be portrayed as "something that occurs 'just in passing,' without ever overemphasizing its importance." Just so, Brueghel's painting dramatizes the continuation of life and shows the fall of the legendary figure as a minor and transitory event. Like the sea that will swallow up the boy without a trace, the world remains undisturbed, and so does the world order. The boy fell in the first place because, venturing too close to the sun, his wings melted: so that the boundaries governing human aspiration, the lines marking "this far and no farther," remain in place. The sun is present in the painting by implication as the source of shadows and the cause of the boy's fall. Along with the well-cultivated earth, with its furrows like ripples or waves, the vast realms of air and water present themselves to the eye. The fourth element, fire, presents itself to the mind's eye. Each of the traditional elements of Nature is accounted for, and each implies the others.

And this vision of a world order that remains intact even in the face of disaster goes back to the beginnings of our literature. In the *Iliad* as Sarpedon, the son of Zeus himself, lies dead on the battlefield, warriors swarm over him

as flies
through a sheepfold thunder about the pails overspilling
milk, in the season of spring when the milk splashes in the
buckets.
So they swarmed over the dead man.

This cannot mean that the carnage of war possesses the loveliness of spring, which would be grotesque, but that the passage of the seasons and the order of life remain blessedly unchanged even in the face of the cataclysm of the Trojan War. In verses like these, a scholar has observed, "Homer is saying that the Trojan War has not encroached upon the lives of all men. Elsewhere the dolphin leap and the shepherds drowse in the peace of the mountains." When the butler's servant, beaming with "the joy of life," attends to his pathetic master in *The Death of Ivan Ilych*, we pick up a similar affirmation of the persistence of life.

BEING ABLE to see over the plowman's shoulder and behind his back, we perceive more than he does; but the truth is that *Landscape with the Fall of Icarus* flatters our feeling of superiority only to delude us. Only because we are informed by the title of the painting do we know of the boy's identity and story. We see no more of his wings than the plowman does of the boy himself. Unless alerted, we might not even recognize his crooked, inverted, disappearing leg as a leg. In brief, if not for the title we would have no idea of what the painting was about. It is anything but transparent. Moreover, the knowledge conveyed by the title is available only after the fact. In real time, while the boy falls from the sky, no one can look up and say, "That is the boy Icarus falling to his death because he ignored his father's warning and soared too close to the sun." Any actual observer would understand no more of the event than Brueghel's plowman, who doesn't even notice it. The plowman doesn't see what we see, but—contrary to earlier impressions—at least he sees for himself instead of having things edited and labeled for him. History itself looks different in retrospect than in prospect, before outcomes are known and labels applied. In the present moment we are subject to the law of ignorance, a condition also built into those great novels that draw us artfully—deliberately but with seeming naturalness—into errors of perception and judgment. While silent on the public issues of the day, Jane Austen reveals what it is to live in time in the first place by entangling the reader in such mistakes.

The cancer patient too abides by the law of ignorance, and gains a heightened sense of the unknown simply by standing in its presence.

THE ICARUS STORY is read as a parable of the quest for forbidden experience, and in that sense forbidden knowledge. To many of the heirs of the Enlightenment, any restriction on knowledge is intolerable. Yet some in the breast cancer world who question the wisdom of mass screening think it may be advisable not to know of cancer—cancer that will never amount to a danger in many cases and is beyond treatment in others. Prostate cancer presents parallel issues, the patient soon finding that the quest for knowledge leads to wildly contradictory medical recommendations, inconsistent numbers, promising mirages, missing data, and visions of mutilation more than the mind can bear: bewilderment, paralysis, and horror.

As we learn from Brueghel's contemporary Montaigne, medicine in that time had not

> reached such certainty that, no matter what we do, we cannot find some authority for doing it. Medicine changes according to the climate, according to the phases of the moon, according to Fernel and according to Scaliger. If your own doctor does not find it good for you to sleep, to use wine or any particular food, do not worry: I will find you another who does not agree with his advice. The range of differing medical arguments and opinions embraces every sort of variety.

While medical opinion on prostate cancer is not such a circus, the understanding of the disease has still not reached the point where factional differences die away. The disease itself seems to call for a spirit of uncertainty in the tradition of Montaigne—not a doubt that withers all possibility of action, but a doubt that convinces you to do what you can within the limits of knowledge, like the plow-man effective within his own limits. And who can say that the plowman is unaware of those limits?

LOOKING AT Brueghel's plowman, we can only assume that this is just what he is: not one who happens to be plowing or who may tomorrow pilot a ship, but one who works the earth from day to day. Though literature abounds with characters at variance with their role—from Chaucer's Prioress, a nun with the manners of a romantic, to Fyodor Pavlovitch Karamazov, a father who forgets his sons, to Leopold Bloom, who beggars his own description as a sales-man—the plowman appears before us as one who is what he does, and this not in the empty sense that we see him only in a plowing capacity. The plowman does his work like an artisan, practically etching the land, and only one who considered his work important, not incidental, to his very identity could do it this well. Dr. Green for his part does not come across as someone who happens to do medicine or really lives to ski. He too is an artisan, and in confer-ring with us on September 12, 2001, he kept true to his craft. (Only later, upon reflection, did I appreciate just how conscientiously Dr. Green kept to medicine. Never did he offer prescriptions for healthy living, theories of causation, nutritional or psychological nostrums, cautions about stress, referrals to support groups, recommendations of massage, yoga, or vitamins, or preachments of any kind. He did not speak of cancer as an opportunity for personal growth. He did not imply that my disease could not be dealt with unless and until I corrected what was wrong with my life.)

I think of Dr. Green as in his own way a faithful plowman,

doing his work well in the face of disaster. The plowman, however, inhabits an order that remains unchanged, and exemplifies that order. The physician belongs to a world changed irreversibly, and by his patience and skill reaffirms order itself. I am reminded of the reflections of Primo Levi on those prisoners in Auschwitz forced to continue their occupation: "tailors, cobblers, carpenters, blacksmiths, bricklayers. [Levi might perhaps have added himself, a chemist.] Such people, resuming their customary activity, recovered at the same time, to some extent, their human dignity." By some means Dr. Green was able to preserve his patient's dignity even when it seemed there was none left to preserve.

Returning the next day to classes that had not met since September 10, I faced the issue of whether to stick to the syllabus or put it aside. Thinking of Dr. Green, I did the first. I held classes as usual—not in the spirit of ignoring disaster but in the desire to rebuild in the face of disaster. Once again I was trying to argue students out of the belief that all of literature is about nothing but indifference to human suffering, and that certain politically special themes come tagged with the literary equivalent of pink ribbons.

BEYOND SHAME AND GUILT

HOW DID Bob Dole, of all people, a Kansas conservative, become a spokesman for Viagra? Going from one campaign to another, the former candidate for president was now the crowned king of impotence. Dole could tell himself that his commercials weren't intended to goad or shock but to help, while Pfizer could tell itself that if it could win over this expressionless heartlander, it could certainly win the American public. Carried out in the name of medicine, the sort of line-crossing that Dole himself might have resented in performance art or *The Vagina Monologues* thus became— tasteful?

Viagra was on my mind during the preparations for surgery, and especially after a conference with my radiation oncologist, Dr. Marion, wherein she spoke to me as no one, woman or man, had ever spoken before. Like her bleached hair and crude puns, Dr. Marion's clinical descriptions and her view of sex as a function I found wonderful, somehow; for she too emits the joy of life. I followed as she went down a painful list of possible complications and side effects, striking them off with a flourish one at a time—and all of this in a becomingly tight skirt. In some cases Viagra is advised after surgery. As forward as she was about these things, though, never did

[*34*]

she, or Dr. Green for that matter, offer advice about how to live with cancer.

A book on prostate cancer written by three physicians and endorsed by the American Cancer Society offers much counsel of that kind, as though in the end medicine dissolved into psychotherapy. "Recognize and Manage Your Emotions." From this book's point of view, shame is something to be overcome—an obstacle to well-being. Among the statements by patients scattered through the text is one by "Jim, a former electrical engineer now living in Washington," who underwent castration.

> "I sometimes say that I'm a steer instead of a bull. But I couldn't talk about it at first. I was as bad as the rest of us men. My attitude was, 'Just clam up. Don't tell anybody anything. It's too embarrassing.' Well, now I say the hell with it. I tell everyone, because I figure I can help somebody get diagnosed earlier."

Behind stories like this in the cancer literature stands the ideal of a person endowed with what Iris Murdoch calls "an empty lonely freedom, a freedom, if he wishes, to 'fly in the face of the facts.' [This freedom is] the fearful solitude of the individual marooned upon a tiny island in the middle of a sea of scientific facts," able to escape only "by a wild leap of the will." The image of a medical castrate proclaiming himself to one and all illustrates very well the pathos of this wild and lonely liberty in the face of science. And finally the purpose served by Jim's proclamations is self-expression. Maybe in some world without conflict, confusion, or irony, where nothing comes between self and others, hearing a tale of castration would move every man to do the rational thing and get screened for prostate cancer (assuming that *is* the rational thing). But in the world we inhabit, some of Jim's audience might be so horrified that they put cancer out of their minds. Others, learning that castration was part of Jim's treatment and not an effect of the disease itself, might reasonably resolve never to enter a doctor's office. For better or worse, we do not live in an age of transparency. Even the cancer "survivors" cited in *Prostate Cancer: What Every Man—and His Family—Needs to Know* are identified, like Jim, by first name only, as though concealment had some place in the world after all.

While cancer once suggested a lack of self-restraint, today the whispered word is that it comes of too much self-restraint: stress. But despite the paradoxical disrepute that shame, concealment, and everything connected with them seem to have fallen into—it is shame, some say, that keeps men from getting checked for prostate cancer—is it really the case that shame as such ought to be abolished as a relic of a dark past, that we have nothing to be ashamed of but shame itself? I question not so much the introduction of private concerns into the public realm (for, in a sense, that goes back at least as long as the modern novel) as the advertising of such acts as a blow struck against ignorance and repression and a de facto contribution to the public good. Even Jim maintains that in baring himself to the world he does good for others. The cult of disclosure doesn't simply ignore the principle that some things "require the cover of privacy to retain their significance and emotional vibrancy," it repudiates it, arguing with much pomp and posture that secrecy of any kind obstructs human well-being and that to make public private things is to perform a daring act of emancipation. A woman displays the scar where her breast was, like an Amazon of the new age. Birth appears on television. But surely, things that Dr. Marion said in private would be tasteless and banal on television. If the ambiguities of thought can't be fitted into the categories of an opinion poll (at least not without flattening and falsification), neither can the most private experiences be made into advertisements of our own emancipation without cost to their own truth and to the public realm itself.

The combined message of Viagra ads, voices of liberation, consciousness-raisers, goads, iconoclasts, therapists, and other movers of opinion is that shame really is a superstition—a survival from the days of irrationality and a fetter on the human capacity for progress. Guilt for its part is considered a blight on happiness and approved only in the form of social conscience. But a guilt that is less a threatening force than an instrument of enlightened policy is guilt in name only. Despite the anthropological distinction between guilt and shame, it seems plain that great changes are at work in our culture in the standards and economy of both. Even without therapeutic taboos on blame, backed up by a kind of instinctive reluctance to judge, guilt would be eroded by our culture's very theme of moving forward, putting the past behind you. Putting the past behind you is the one thing guilt will not permit. The Ancient Mariner relives his crime. From a progressive point of view, there must be something wrong with a force that keeps you so painfully stuck in the past. Like Hamlet refusing to let go of his grief and accept a new tender of paternal love, the guilty one remains tied to yesterday and perversely, neurotically resists the flow of time. Progressively speaking, the ideal form of guilt may be survivor guilt, precisely because the sufferer has done nothing to earn it. Survivor guilt is guilt without anything to be guilty of, a demonstration as it were of the baseless nature of guilt itself. Both in breast and prostate cancer literature you occasionally come across a profession of guilt over having survived a disease others died of. Also acceptable, in this case because the guilty one has done nothing but behave like someone with a social conscience, is the guilt of the physician who does everything he can to move minority men to get screened for prostate cancer, but with poor results. The physician feels remorse not for what he has done but for the history of oppression that makes these men suspicious of the medical profession. He feels remorse, as it were, for what others have done.

With the exception of the sort of admirably innocent guilt of these examples, guilt is considered a product of social conditioning and associated with backward notions. Some think of guilt as a kind of cancer in its own right, destroying well-being, consuming us from within. Guilt seems particularly out of step with the utilitarianism that supplies modernity's prevailing philosophy. If a utilitarian like Jeremy Bentham wants to establish an economy, a sort of rational minimum, of punishment, there is something distinctly irrational in the mode of punishment called guilt that goes on and on after the offense itself has become a memory, again as in the case of the Ancient Mariner. To some, guilt itself may represent an offense to progress. Recent testimony in Washington by the leading proponent of prostate cancer research in the United States—a man who put a notorious past behind him—yielded hints of what lies beyond guilt and shame.

ON JUNE 16, 1999, Michael Milken, the founder, president, and chairman of the Association for the Cure of Cancer of the Prostate (CaP CURE) pleaded with a Senate subcommittee for increased funding for research.

> The federal investment in finding cures for cancer—$3 billion annually—is less than 0.0004% of our gross domestic product,

or about one-seventh of what Americans spend on beauty products. At the same time, we often hear that our nation is spending more than $100 billion annually—much of it by the federal government—for cancer *care*. With the graying of the baby-boom generation and its greater risk of cancer as members pass the age of 50, cancer-care dollars are likely to double within a decade. Is there any organization that would spend more than 35 times as much to deal with the effects of a problem as it would to solve the problem? It makes no sense in the private sector, and, with current concerns about spending rates and budget caps, it should make no sense in government. . . .

In the six years since my diagnosis, the federal government has invested about $800 million to find a cure for prostate cancer, only about $3,000 for each life lost to the disease. Compare that to the nearly $3 billion our government has wisely appropriated during that six-year period for breast cancer research—a disease that annually claims approximately the same number of lives. Or compare it to the more than $10 billion that the federal government has spent trying to find a cure for AIDS. It's not that breast cancer research or AIDS research gets too much research funding. As long as lives are lost to those diseases, or pain and suffering endured, no amount is "too much." It's just that prostate cancer research has gotten too little.

So the speech continues, an impassioned plea and in part a cogent one. In part, because the sort of economic arguments marshaled by Milken in favor of an all-out assault on prostate cancer have also been marshaled against the overtreatment of the disease. In the minds of many, it doesn't make economic sense to throw everything we have at a disease that can often be left to itself. Milken's counter, that as long as lives are lost to disease no expense can be too much, is unconvincing. Are we to invest the national treasury in the quest for eternal life? Icarus crossed a limit. We too are subject to limits, first and last, but not exclusively, those imposed by mortality. In a finite world, money spent on one thing cannot be spent on another—in fact money going to one form of cancer research cannot go to another. No doubt Milken doesn't wish to subtract funds from breast cancer or AIDS research but to increase funding vastly for all such research in keeping with his rhetoric of all-out effort and his principle that no expenditure can be too much—but in the world as it is given to us, this cannot be. If, as he projects, "the future liability of prostate cancer is, in fact, in the *trillions* of dollars" (his emphasis), it would be only prudent to lay out a trillion or two right now by way of prevention. Such prudence is not of this world. So too, the vision of a full-scale war against the real enemy, cancer, has the exorbitance of a modest proposal. "Consider," Milken says,

> what part of our national income we have spent on the military in wartime, and then consider the fact that an American soldier is more likely to die from cancer than from enemy action. Just as we don't fight guns-and-bullets wars with a 40-hour week, we must recognize that the war against the foreign invader we call cancer is a 24-hour-a-day, seven-day-a-week effort.

Like much cancer rhetoric, only more emphatically, Milken's argument assumes an audience that is in denial of the glaringly obvious, that needs to have its mind thrown open like a shutter; and perhaps that is just what is wrong with the argument.

Not only is there no reason to believe that the members of

Congress are locked in a collective state of denial, but the case for some sort of total war on cancer is not as obvious as the rhetoric makes out. For one thing, the rhetoric assumes that the nation will be spared actual wars. Additionally, as noted, the numbers themselves cut two ways. Even mass screening for prostate (or breast) cancer is criticized on the ground that at some point the cost of all those tests becomes vastly excessive. Maybe it is to trump arguments like this that Milken uses such astronomical numbers. "Prostate cancer will affect about one man in six in this country, which means that more than six million boomers could become its victims during the next decades resulting in more than $600 billion in expenditures." Under the guise of rational calculation, such rhetoric makes calculation itself meaningless. As in Swift's "Modest Proposal," which is also dressed in numbers, there is a fantastic, runaway quality to Milken's appeal, and beyond this a vast immodesty. Swift's speaker keeps his name to himself even as he imagines a monument to himself in the public square as a benefactor of humanity. Milken comes before the Senate subcommittee as a crusader on behalf of humanity and a voice of social conscience, not mentioning a criminal record that cannot have been unknown to his audience.

In the 1980s, as an executive of Drexel Burnham Lambert, Michael Milken pioneered the use of junk bonds to finance new ventures and corporate takeovers. In 1989 he was indicted for securities fraud and racketeering, and in the next year, following a plea bargain, was sentenced to ten years in federal prison. He served twenty-two months and paid a fine of some hundreds of millions of dollars. In the manner of the tycoon turned public benefactor, he established CaP CURE in 1993, the same year he was released from prison and diagnosed with advanced prostate cancer. (Later Milken fell afoul of the Securities and Exchange Commission once again.)

In spite of his guilty plea, Milken seems to deny his guilt, stating in his "biography" that the violations he was charged with "before his case had not been subject to criminal prosecution." His good works do look like an attempt at expiation, but on the other hand a guilt that can be used at will and directed to constructive social ends, a guilt that is putty in one's hands, has already lost some of the un-tamed power of guilt itself.

When they send you to prison they don't take away your right to speak, but someone who had gone to prison for fraud might hes-itate to lecture the United States Senate if that person had a keen sense of shame. In Milken's presentation of himself as a voice of simple economic prudence there is something especially brazen, seeing that in the one year of 1987 he earned $550 million. Finan-cially speaking, Michael Milken is the man in the moon. Having lost relatives to cancer and having had the disease himself, Milken may have felt that cancer takes precedence over everything else, and that his new mission obliterates the dishonor of his past. He comes before the Senate, therefore, as one born again, his criminal record washed away in his new identity as a cancer survivor and crusader. But in the rhetoric of the new Milken there remains something of the old Milken—an inordinancy, a kind of zeal for the infinite, a will to shatter existing practices. Swift's proposer is marooned on a tiny island of self in the middle of a sea of facts; Milken proposes to conquer cancer by a national leap of the will. When he calculates the economic value of lives lost to cancer each year—at $4 million per life, "the 560,000 individuals who will die from cancer this year result in losses in *trillions*"—he speaks unmistakably in the manner of the "Modest Proposal" with its estimates of the economic value of the human yearling. But, again, the real resemblance between the two speakers, Swift's humble visionary and Michael Milken, lies in a vast lack of modesty.

Says Swift's figure in closing,

> I profess, in the sincerity of my heart, that I have not the least personal interest in endeavoring to promote this necessary work, having no other motive than the public good of my country, by advancing our trade, providing for infants, relieving the poor, and giving some pleasure to the rich.

Similarly claiming high motives, Michael Milken in 1996 declared, "I have never been motivated by money in my entire life." Milken's "biography," presumably authorized if not written by himself, identifies him as one of the world's biggest givers ("behind Bill Gates and ahead of the Rockefeller brothers") and credits him with advancing cancer research "by 40 years." But even as a financier, it appears, Milken was a benefactor of humanity. "Milken is often said to have revolutionized modern capital markets," writes Milken, "making them more efficient, dynamic and democratic" as well as making possible "America's explosion of wealth and creativity during the 1990s." His innovations are responsible for the creation of "millions of jobs." "In 1996, *Fortune* magazine called him 'a genius.'" (In fact the September 30, 1996, issue of *Fortune* takes a two-sided view of Milken, casting particular irony on his efforts as publicist for himself and redeemer of his own reputation.) Whether he is advancing our trade, as Swift puts it, or promoting cancer research, it seems that Michael Milken possesses the zeal of a visionary, a drive to push limits, and a way of getting into the headlines. I am particularly struck by Milken's all-but-voiced claim to have reduced prostate cancer deaths in the United States. "Since CaP CURE was founded, annual U.S. prostate cancer deaths have declined from 43,000 to 31,500 even as the population most at risk—men over 50—grew substantially because of aging baby boomers." From what I have seen, good medical practice follows a different path from Milken's: it is subtle and at times uncertain, not grandiose and inflated, and its practitioners do not advertise themselves or set themselves up as preservers of the nation.

Displayed in Dr. Marion's office *were* press clippings—not of herself as a fighter in the war against cancer but of her father, a fighter pilot during the Korean War. In a great glass case mounted on the wall were the aviator's jacket, scarf, and medals, as well as yellowing newspaper articles about his exploits. Dr. Marion took particular pride in pointing out a chunk of metal. "That's shrapnel taken from his leg."

IT WAS Swift's mighty opposite Locke who best set forth the ideal of "a human agent who is able to remake himself by methodical and disciplined action": the ideal of changing oneself by changing one's habits. In spite of the unlikeliness of the notion of shedding one's character, and the oddity of being at once the manager of this change and the entity being changed, few seem willing to question the project of remaking ourselves from the inside out by some sort of therapeutic program. In the case of Michael Milken, that program involved the adoption of a new diet as well as meditation, herbal therapy, and aromatherapy, all in an effort to rid himself of cancer. He also underwent radiation and hormone treatments. This much is clear: few can have invested more than Milken in the project of self-transformation, yet the old Milken remains.

The evangelist for cancer research who came before the United

States Senate bears a strange resemblance to the disgraced financier whose story was once all over the press but now went unmentioned. It is not just that his plea to the Senate deals in impossibly large numbers and defends increased funding for prostate research on the grounds that "the value of the investment is already assured." As one of a number of innovative funding mechanisms (like junk-bond financing in its time), Milken proposed the sale of "cancer war bonds." Did the senators wince when they heard Milken talking up bonds all over again? Perhaps they didn't take up the idea of cancer war bonds because they didn't wish to invest in a metaphor. Perhaps the alternative therapies in which Milken takes an interest seemed to them junk science, by analogy with junk bonds. But perhaps too they didn't want to be seen to be rehabilitating the reputation of Michael Milken by applying to the cause of medical research the same kind of creativity the financier brought to his work in the 1980s.

THE BREAST AND
THE PROSTATE

NO SOONER did Dr. Green call to report cancer than he recommended removal of the prostate. He isn't the directive kind, though, and in our conference of September 12 radical surgery was talked of as one option, nothing more. Once seeds were looked into, my wife Lizzie and I decided on the spot—seeing no need to draw things out further—for seeds and not surgery, a decision endorsed by Dr. Green as if he had never advised the other course at all. While irradiating the prostate from within is said to kill cancer cells and spare healthy ones, it is still a nonspecific treatment destined one day to seem crude. Like horses threading needles in *Gulliver's Travels,* it works, more or less, but lacks finesse. Still, compared to the brute-force tactic of removing the prostate from the body, it has a lot to recommend it. As I looked back later over our decision against radical surgery, I thought of breast cancer patients who once would have undergone such surgery themselves but now received less devastating treatments. The two diseases—prostate cancer and breast cancer—indeed have much in common.

IN THE CASE of both prostate and breast cancer, the wisdom of aggressive screening has been questioned, meaning that those confronting these cancers, either in fact or in prospect, are up against a disease more subtle than our instruments of detection and in some ways still beyond the reach and understanding of medicine. In neither case can dangerous cancers be distinguished from indolent ones at an early stage. Both prostate and breast cancer patients come face to face with the discouraging possibility that biology really is destiny. Both communities learn to their sorrow just how fallacious the myth is that we have entered the promised land of medical knowledge. Men who inherit a mutant gene associated with breast cancer stand a higher risk of prostate cancer. In both cancers, it seems, evidence of the disease shows up in autopsies of those who died of other causes. In Japan, rates for both diseases run lower than in the United States. Two or three years before my diagnosis, a neighbor two or three years older was struck with breast cancer. Both cancers are "amongst the most malignant and clinically intransigent" form of the disease. Like mirror conditions, prostate and breast cancer are diagnosed in about the same numbers and account for about the same number of deaths per year in this country.

Writes a critic of mammography,

> While mammography . . . does detect some potentially deadly cancers and has thus saved some women's lives, it also picks up many times more cancers that would never have become symptomatic during the patient's lifetime. . . . Thus, for every woman saved by early diagnosis, many others receive costly, painful, and potentially dangerous treatment to destroy tumors

that pose little or no threat—tumors that they might die *with*,
not *of.*

Substitute PSA and prostate cancer for mammography and breast
cancer and the passage loses nothing. Both diseases pose a kind of
humiliating conundrum to human intelligence. "Die with and not
of" is in fact a prostate cancer tag line. As children we think of the
other sex as another world. Later we receive the revelations of sex
itself. Later still our bodies seem to tell us of the kinship, deep
down, of men and women.

In addition to the biological resemblances between prostate
and breast cancer, similar conventions have sprung up around these
diseases. Both prostate and breast cancer have interest groups, publicity mechanisms, buttons, pins, press kits, a support culture, a
rhetoric. The diseases have been blanketed with institutions. Moreover, each disease has a constituency, and within each group some
feel disadvantaged with respect to the other. Men point to the un-
derfunding of prostate cancer research as against breast cancer and
AIDS. (Thus, for example, Michael Milken compares the $800 mil-
lion in federal funds committed to prostate research from 1993 to
1999 to "the nearly $3 billion our government has wisely appropri-
ated during that six-year period for breast cancer research—a disease that annually claims approximately the same number of lives.")
Alleging reverse sexism, a Toronto physician argues that "an active
70-year-old woman would never be asked to forgo treatment for her
breast cancer. Seventy-year-old men with prostate cancer often are.
They are told to wait—for another disease." Some women, however,
contend that medical research and clinical trials favor men and that
breast cancer is itself underfunded as against prostate cancer. A
breast cancer activist argues that "As long as people pretend that

there is a cure for breast cancer, women will continue to die from neglect of this disease," as if the same couldn't be said of prostate cancer. In designating October as Breast Cancer Awareness Month and November as Prostate Cancer Awareness Month, it is as though a parental government were making a point of showing no favoritism as between squabbling children. The Postal Service is said to be preparing a Prostate Cancer stamp to go along with the Breast Cancer stamp already issued.

Historically women have had it worse than men, but I think it can be said that in poetry and art the breast has it over the prostate. The breast is an image of loveliness:

> Thy two breasts are like two young roes that are twins, which feed among the lilies. . . .
> Thou art all fair, my love; there is no spot in thee. (Song of Solomon, 4:5, 7)

Again:

> Thy stature is like to a palm tree, and thy breasts to clusters of grapes.
> I said, I will go up to the palm tree, I will take hold of the boughs thereof: now also thy breasts shall be as clusters of the vine, and the smell of thy nose like apples. (Song of Solomon, 7:7–8)

Says Marvell's speaker, addressing his coy mistress: "An hundred years should go to praise / Thine eyes, and on thy forehead gaze; / Two hundred to adore each breast." The prostate does not seem to have as many admirers as the breast, and many cultures have come and gone on this earth that knew nothing of its existence. Only in

[49]

the eighteenth century was the gland identified. May I not live to read poems to the prostate.

Next to its counterpart, prostate cancer has blessedly little public relations value. The glamour industry that sponsors breast cancer events has left prostate cancer to itself for now, nor does the men's disease yet have its own civic festivals and occasions of organized happiness. Dulling the image of prostate cancer still further is its reputation as a disease of old men—and a boring disease at that, something men die with and not of, an ailment of age in a world abashed by age itself.

THE IDEA that some things might be too profound to be spoken, some experiences too private to advertise, has been rejected with a vengeance in the world of the pink ribbon. As Barbara Ehrenreich writes in her reflection on the culture of breast cancer,

> You can dress in pink-beribboned sweatshirts, denim shirts, pajamas, lingerie, aprons, loungewear, shoelaces, and socks; accessorize with pink rhinestone brooches, angel pins, scarves, caps, earrings, and bracelets; brighten up your home with breast-cancer candles, stained-glass pink-ribbon candleholders, coffee mugs, pendants, wind chimes, and night-lights; pay your bills with special BreastChecks or a special line of Checks for the Cure. "Awareness" beats secrecy and stigma of course, but I can't help noticing that the existential space in which a friend has earnestly advised to me "confront [my] mortality" bears a striking resemblance to the mall.

Not his cloak or even his tears can denote Hamlet truly, but the world of cancer tokens knows no such problems of representation, and things you might expect to find in a gift shop in Disney-land become signifiers of remembrance and hope. The effect of all the teddy bears and pink trinkets, Barbara Ehrenreich believes, is to infantilize the patient. "You are encouraged to regress to a little-girl state, to suspend critical judgment, and to accept whatever measures the doctors, as parent surrogates, choose to accept." Only women are so demeaned. If Michael Milken, among others, finds prostate research at a disadvantage with respect to its sister cause, Barbara Ehrenreich finds women themselves at a disadvantage to men. "Certainly men diagnosed with prostate cancer do not receive gifts of Matchbox cars."

Even theories of cancer come pink and blue. That "women migrating to industrialized countries quickly develop the same breast-cancer rates as those who are native born" Barbara Ehrenreich, like others, construes as a sign of environmental causation. And within the category of "environment" she does not include diet, alleging that any dietary contribution to breast cancer has been "largely ruled out." In the prostate cancer literature you find the argument that immigrants from nations with a low incidence of the disease soon catch up to the American average—and that this effect marks the influence of diet. The immigrants, or their children, are starting to eat like Americans and getting sick accordingly. Theories of environmental causation advanced by critics like Barbara Ehrenreich ought to apply in the case of prostate cancer (men too being exposed to pesticides and other toxins), and the claims about diet made in the prostate literature ought to apply to breast cancer (women too being under the dominion of "the Western diet"), yet the arguments ignore each other. Barbara Ehrenreich rises to indignation at something she calls the Cancer Industrial Complex, that is, the corporations said to be responsible for cancer (a vision shared by many who take their own ideological fervor for a finding of science). If women somehow brought breast cancer on themselves by a bad diet, there would be no one to be indignant at. Men, for their part, mostly lacking any conception of their group as an oppressed class, are better served by the argument that they are poisoning themselves. The exception to this rule is suggestive. In the case of black Americans, who are at markedly higher risk for prostate cancer, the publicity about the disease stays away from the issue of diet, presumably because no one wants to be seen blaming a historically oppressed group for its own plight. The general importance of diet is noted, as is the high rate of prostate cancer among black Americans, but for ideological reasons the two topics are kept well apart. Of the two contradictory arguments cited above—one in favor of environmental causation to the exclusion of diet, the other in favor of diet to the exclusion of the environment—each has also been fashioned to meet the ideological requirements of its maker.

ACCORDING TO Barbara Ehrenreich, the infantilization of women at the hands of the breast cancer industry is a throwback to the era of "patriarchal medicine." Here then is another example of pushing against a door already open. The very radiologist mentioned in the author's second paragraph, an authority who "never has the courtesy to show her face," is a woman. A patriarchal woman? My own radiation oncologist, also a woman, was patriarchal in no respect; nor was I encouraged either by her or Dr. Green to abandon judgment and place myself in their hands. (On the contrary: Dr. Marion considered a promotional video on seed implants to be an insult to critical intelligence.) That women are the special victims of the Cancer Industrial Complex, a variant of the Military-Industrial

Complex, is itself a fable that inhibits critical judgment. Nevertheless there *is* something regressive about the ever-growing concern with health. Two weeks after surgery this was brought home to me by a campus newsletter—an in-house publication that once carried information about faculty achievements—with a pink-ribbon theme.

Bearing the headline, "Breast Cancer Impacts Campus Employees," the newsletter featured the story of a worker in the audit department being treated for breast cancer. "Every day she wears a quilted pink-ribbon pin made for her by a friend. . . . 'Sometimes,' she says, 'it's the little things that help the most—like prayers and positive thoughts and pink ribbons.'" Reminded that October is Breast Cancer Awareness Month, readers are asked to wear the pink ribbon attached to the newsletter itself "to help raise awareness and show support for [the audit worker] and other campus colleagues battling the disease." Although my university does not observe Prostate Cancer Awareness Month, or not yet, the disease has its own awareness crusades, rhetoric of battle, campaigns against shame, and support culture. In effect it has its own ribbon, as if its very seriousness had called forth the most trivial formulas of consolation. Ivan Ilych finds the "awful, solemn" act of his own death degraded to the level of chitchat. The prostate cancer patient finds that the event that has taken hold of him actually has its own conventions, conventions very like those of the pink ribbon attached to the newsletter. I imagine that before long, prostate cancer will evolve its own equivalent of BreastChecks and thematic coffee mugs. As to the campus newsletter, it contains not a single academic feature and barely an academic note. In addition to the front-page article on breast cancer, it does contain, however, paragraphs on End-of-Life Care, the Flu Shootout, the Blue Cross pharmacy plan, Fear of

Speaking, and Winter Fitness, as well as a note on a Wellness class entitled "Moving On," which I thought meant getting over grief and breakups but turns out to refer to fitness.

The story of the boy Icarus ignoring his father's admonition, flying too close to the sun and falling to his death, warns against defying limits. In the runaway expansion of health concerns our culture has evolved a new style of excess, as the "cornucopia" of breast cancer goods cited by Barbara Ehrenreich, from sweatshirts to wind chimes, is itself a catalogue of excess. In the spirit of true limitlessness, this expansion takes in not just bodily but mental health.

> In the 1950s, it was thought that only fifty people per million were depressed. Nowadays no one blinks on being told that depression affects over 100,000 per million and that it leads to more disability and economic disadvantage than any other disorder.

This makes the thousandfold increase in the frequency of obsessive-compulsive disorder seem modest by contrast, though perhaps the real obsession is the drive to keep up with pharmaceutical advances and the devouring preoccupation with health itself. I doubt that the corporations created cancer, but that we ourselves, with their encouragement, have fashioned new ailments I have no doubt at all. Mr. Woodhouse in *Emma* can tolerate only a thin gruel and talks of nothing but his nerves, the danger of drafts, and his and others' delicacy: a kindly but infantile man who has to be treated as a child by his own daughter. Like a Dickens character, Mr. Woodhouse imprisons himself within a fiction of his own making, a victim of his imagination. But in a sense he really is sick. If, as it used to be said, health is unconscious of itself, then an endless fixation on health constitutes a loss of well-being in its own right. A wag observes that many lives could be saved if only "all men had their prostates removed at age 50 and if all women had their breasts removed at age 50." Health can be purchased at the price of health itself.

If Icarus is childish in his blind craving for independence—of his father and of his world's laws—the therapeutic culture glimpsed in my university's newsletter promotes an excessive dependence.

Some years before John Stuart Mill warned of a tyranny that did not employ the power of the state, Tocqueville prophesied that a new, soft despotism would spring from the soil of American equality. Over the citizenry would arise

> an immense and tutelary power, which takes upon itself alone to secure their gratifications and to watch over their fate. That power is absolute, minute, regular, provident, and mild. It would be like the authority of a parent if, like that authority, its object was to prepare men for manhood; but it seeks, on the contrary, to keep them in perpetual childhood. . . . It provides for their security, foresees and supplies their necessities, facilitates their pleasures, [and] manages their principal concerns.

What Tocqueville has in mind is an overmanaging state, but his words apply with strange accuracy to the helping community—extending beyond doctors and nurses to therapists, facilitators, nutritionists, grief counselors, addiction specialists, workshop leaders, Fear of Speaking authorities, social workers, tutors, mentors, advocates, and a hundred others ready at all times to relieve our anxieties and, in the name of care, take into their velvet hands our principal concerns. Tocqueville foresees a new power at once "absolute, regular, minute, provident, and mild." The president of the university—a man with the temperament of a monarch but the politics of a strict progressive—once sent a Christmas memo to the campus reminding everyone to wear galoshes. But what if a mild state of well-being could be provided in regular chemical doses? Of Bentham and James Mill it has been said that "if anyone had offered them a medicine which could scientifically be shown to put those who took it into a state of permanent contentment, their premises would have bound them to accept this as the panacea for all that they thought evil." In the era of Prozac, things have progressed beyond the stage of the thought-experiment.

Perhaps the childishness fostered by a caring system so deep-reaching, so provident, and so mild contributes to the whining tone of our public debate. The "culture of complaint" is supported by the culture of health complaints. Complaint anyway seems to be regarded as the supreme mode of argument. Says Mrs. Bennet in *Pride and Prejudice,* "Those who do not complain are never pitied." Men point to the funding of breast-cancer research; women contend that research favors men and that they themselves are the victims of patriarchal medicine. To match the pink ribbon, some in the prostate-cancer world actually use the blue-ribbon emblem. Instinctively, as it were, the factions revert to the colors of the nursery. (Some recommend that doctors post their own baby pictures in their office.) *Us Too!*, the name of a prominent organization of prostate cancer patients, comes very close to the child's "Me too!" Over the quarreling parties stands a government which, like a fair-minded, Tocquevillian parent, gives women the month of October and men November. Politically speaking, complaint does some good; but those in suffering and those who do any good work at all know that complaint does no good.

THE EXPERIENCE of the mammogram—like the PSA test for men, an unreliable instrument of detection and a subject of controversy—is described by Barbara Ehrenreich, in part:

> Sometimes the machine doesn't work, and I get squished into position to no purpose at all. More often, the X ray is successful but apparently alarming to the invisible radiologist, off in some remote office, who calls the shots and never has the courtesy to show her face with an apology or an explanation.

It is as though some medical prison had come into being, an impression reinforced when the author speaks of herself as a "suspect" and mammography as an instrument of cancer "surveillance." In the notorious Panopticon of Jeremy Bentham, an inspector keeps inmates under surveillance from his own position of concealment. And this asymmetry is matched by another: the inspector (Bentham himself) acts from higher motives than any his wards are familiar with. Although Dr. Marion, the radiation oncologist, certainly had me mapped out, her relation to me was not of this kind. She never acted like a higher being.

As she once revealed with a kind of mock embarrassment, Dr. Marion studied animal science before moving into medicine, a history that may have something to do with her view of the human animal. Her manner is brash but in a way that you find affirmative, even joyful—a good thing in a cancer doctor. There is something of the rodeo queen, and nothing of the pink ribbon, in Dr. Marion.

As I was being readied for surgery, Dr. Marion came by to introduce herself to Lizzie and say a few friendly words. For some reason she took off her surgical cap and shook her hair out, and there came into view a pair of smart diamond earrings. The rest is blurry, except that a nurse mentioned that Dr. Marion herself would undergo surgery the next day.

Later I learned it was breast reconstruction surgery. I did not learn from her. Whether out of pride or the sort of professional detachment that Ivan Ilych himself specializes in, whether out of a care to keep the patient and not herself at the center of things or simply because it did not pertain to her treatment of me, Dr. Marion—who spoke with such zest about the male condition—never once mentioned her own state.

THE CORRESPONDENCE between breast and prostate cancer, extending even to the conventions and rhetoric that surround these conditions, can change one's view of sexual differences. Psychologists muse on the feminine side of men, literary theorists on androgyny and cross-dressing in Shakespeare, philosophers employ a generic "she" in place of, or alternately with, the masculine pronoun. According to the philosopher Richard Rorty, sensitive moderns like these learn to include formerly alien groups into the category of those like themselves.

> The right way to take the slogan "We have obligations to human beings simply as such" is as a means of reminding ourselves to keep trying to expand our sense of "us" as far as we can. The slogan urges . . . the inclusion among "us" of the family in the next cave, then of the tribe across the river, then of the tribal confederation beyond the mountains, then of the unbelievers beyond the seas (and, perhaps last of all, of the menials who, all this time, have been doing our dirty work).

However, says Rorty, the resemblances among "us" are grounded in nothing in nature; they spring solely from our desire not to be cruel. They reflect well on ourselves but reflect nothing outside ourselves. Human solidarity is not "something that exists antecedently to our recognition of it." The prostate cancer patient offers a kind of experiential dissent. As the patient goes from a state of walking bewilderment to some comprehension of his condition, as he begins to pay attention to cancer, as the resemblances between breast and prostate cancer dawn on him, eventually to grow into something like twinship, as the image of women as another nation turns to dust within him, he acquires the sense that human solidarity is just what Richard Rorty says it is not: something given by nature and waiting to be registered by human perception.

CONSPIRACY OF SILENCE

All profound things, and emotions of things are pre-
ceded and attended by Silence. . . . Silence is the general
consecration of the universe. Silence is the invisible
laying on of the Divine Pontiff's hands upon the world.
Silence is at once the most harmless and the most awful
thing in all nature. It speaks of the Reserved Forces of
Fate. Silence is the only Voice of our God.

—Herman Melville, *Pierre*

WHEN THE embattled protagonist of Tillie Olsen's
"Tell Me a Riddle" (1961) is discovered to have terminal cancer, her
family conspires to keep the truth from her. "She was not to know."
Though supposedly for the dying woman's benefit, this attempt at
deception really springs from the family's own craven hypocrisy and
need for fictions, or so the author implies. Throughout, Eva, the
dying woman, is portrayed as nobler and stronger, endowed with
greater passion, greater fortitude, and greater sympathy with humanity than those closest to her. The sort of deception that recommends itself so naturally to her husband and children, she herself
disdains. In effect the author has used cancer to ennoble the hero-

ine at others' expense. In life, however, reluctance to speak of cancer is not necessarily a proof of hypocrisy and baseness.

AROUND THE TIME I graduated from high school, not long after the publication of "Tell Me a Riddle," the mothers of two friends died—of what, one did not ask. By now breast cancer has come into the open. Considering the effects of treatment, a woman with breast cancer may not be able to help defying the customs of appearance if she intends to be seen in public at all. Recently I came across an acquaintance shuffling two blocks from home in a state of exhaustion. In chemotherapy, she had the head of Gandhi, wizened and bald. That she appeared so in public—striking others with pity and fear—did not seem to give her the thrill of pushing boundaries.

Looking back on the days when cancer was whispered of and those who suffered and died from it were not commemorated, many speak of a conspiracy of silence, as though reticence were an insidious plot, perhaps as insidious as cancer itself. "Silence like a cancer grows." Even now activists of many kinds come forward as shatterers of inhibition and speakers of things dreaded and denied, pretending that others hadn't already done the same thing and that every possible restriction of expression hadn't been under challenge for some time. Our culture has a lot invested in the caricature of the past as a dark house of repression. There is a story abroad that the Victorians would not refer to the breast of a chicken. Whether this is true I don't know, but it is certainly true that the Victorians have served as an ideal straw man—that is, a convenient symbol of hypocrisies and errors from which their successors have been emancipated. In historical fact, the attack on the Victorians has been going forward for a good century now, with the same poses of daring, the same arguments about the salutary effects of shock, and the same assaults on an alleged conspiracy of silence. A chapter of Rochelle Gurstein's study, *The Repeal of Reticence,* is entitled "The Defeat of the 'Conspiracy of Silence.'" It refers to a concerted revolt against reticence launched by the avant-garde of opinion in "the first quarter of the twentieth century." It was at this time that the virtual inventor and certainly the wizard of American public relations, Freud's nephew Edward Bernays, got his start by stirring up public discussion of venereal disease. Were Bernays alive today, he would regard pink-ribbon campaigns as a triumph of organization and public consciousness-raising, the very fruitation of his own technique.

Ironically, the pose of the breaker of taboos seems to require you to ignore your predecessors in defiance. And yet if the critique of the past hadn't already been reduced to a convention, the violation of taboos might not have become such an established practice and might not be so well received. In the very practices of defiance there is something of the comfort of familiarity. Shock itself has its rituals. Even Barbara Ehrenreich's polemic against the Breast Cancer Complex revives an earlier argument—Herbert Marcuse's diatribe against the Military-Industrial Complex in *One-Dimensional Man,* one of the manuals of radicalism in the 1960s. Says Marcuse of the Happy Consciousness generated in American society:

> This sort of well-being, the productive superstructure over the unhappy base of society, permeates the "media" which mediate between the masters and their dependents. Its publicity agents

shape the universe of communication in which the one-dimensional behavior expresses itself. Its language testifies to . . . the systematic promotion of positive thinking and doing, to the concerted attack on transcendent, critical notions.

In Barbara Ehrenreich's Anglicized version, the productive superstructure becomes the corporations producing carcinogens on the one hand and cancer medicines on the other (a double game illustrating Marcuse's contention that the one-dimensional society normalizes contradiction itself). Unhappiness becomes cancer; publicity, Breast Cancer Awareness; positive thinking, the cult of the pink ribbon; and critical notions, those of the author herself. If the earlier argument hadn't already been in place, would the later argument have the shape and the resonance it does? But of course history doesn't begin in the 1960s either. The argument that the cause of disease lies in our way of life (in the case of breast cancer, that of an advanced industrial society) goes back at least to Rousseau's indictment of the most advanced societies of his time:

> If you consider the anguish of mind which consumes us, the violent passions which exhaust and grieve us, the excessive labours with which the poor are overburdened, and the even more dangerous laxity to which the rich abandon themselves, so that the former die of their needs while the latter of their excesses; if you think of the monstrous mixtures they eat, their pernicious seasonings, their corrupt foods and adulterated drugs; the cheating of those who sell such things and the mistakes of those who administer them, of the poison in the vessels used for cooking; if you take note of the epidemic dis-

eases engendered by the bad air where multitudes of men are gathered together, take note also of those occasioned by the delicacy of our way of life . . . you will see how dearly nature makes us pay for the contempt we have shown for her lessons.

But how can a cause of disease so sensationally obvious go unnoticed? Only as a result of some grand deception. At least as Rousseau shades it, the social theory of disease is already an incipient conspiracy theory.

If the many who pose as violators of the conspiracy of silence ask us to forget that the silence has long since been broken, Rousseau's way of shattering the previous limits of expression and performing an act of revelation without precedent or example is enough to make us forget Montaigne. Rousseau's autobiography begins:

> I have resolved on an enterprise which has no precedent, and which, once complete, will have no imitator. My purpose is to display to my kind a portrait in every way true to nature, and the man I shall portray will be myself.

The ideal of living in a world where everything can be shown and everything can be said mirrors Rousseau's obsession with transparency. (Says Rousseau of himself, characteristically: "His heart, transparent as crystal, can hide nothing of what goes on inside.") More disturbingly, the image of the truth-teller challenging a conspiracy of silence mirrors Rousseau's image of himself as the victim of a sinister conspiracy.

Beginning his autobiography in openness of heart, Rousseau ends it beleaguered by enemies who have closed their hearts to him.

> Even to-day, when I can see the most baleful and terrifying plot that has ever been hatched against a man's memory advancing unchecked towards its execution, I shall die a great deal more peacefully, in the certainty that I am leaving behind me in my writings a witness in my favour that will sooner or later triumph over the machinations of men.

Incapable of concealment and wishing to follow only the dictates of his heart, Rousseau finds himself the victim of a conspiracy of the insincere. When cancer polemicists refer to "the medical establishment," they too call up a conspiracy of the insincere. Also in the tradition of Rousseau, Barbara Ehrenreich begins her reflections on breast cancer with the rhetoric of innocence slandered, rhetoric now used with an ironic squint.

> The results of [an] earlier session had aroused some "concern" on the part of the radiologist and her confederate, the gynecologist, so I am back now in the role of a suspect, eager to clear my name, alert to medical missteps and unfair allegations.

Like Rousseau, who also sought to clear his name, the author must contend with a hostile confederacy. Indeed, her essay follows the same trajectory as Rousseau's narrative, beginning with self-revelation and the rhetoric of saying what had never before (at least until recently) been spoken, and terminating in dark speculations about multinational corporations poisoning the world with cancer and making women their dupes. If Rousseau "wills himself the victim of the cruelest possible persecution," the better to establish his innocence and convict his enemies, those who point to the corporations as the cause of cancer invent a persecution still more cruel than anything Rousseau dreamed of. In the Ehrenreich essay, the term "confederate" grows over the pages into a full-blown vision of conspiracy; or as we might say, a Rousseauvian outcry against falsity becomes in the end, as if by sheer momentum, a Rousseauvian vision of cunning forces working in concert—cunning in that the same corporate complex responsible for "doling out" cancer to women underwrites Breast Cancer Awareness.

> What sustained me through the "treatments" is a purifying rage, a resolve, framed in the sleepless nights of chemotherapy, to see the last polluter, along with, say, the last smug health-insurance operator, strangled with the last pink ribbon.

Though not one to take comfort from a breast-cancer teddy bear, the author does find satisfaction in setting fire to straw men. In the real world purifying rage reveals itself as the purging of enemies, the "cleansing" of communities, the drive to eradicate that was witnessed in the emptying of the city of Phnom Penh in the 1970s, eradication being the only way to make sure of getting every last offender.

A scholar notes that Rousseau "almost always attaches [negative value] to whatever is *hidden* or *mysterious*. In all his writing . . . mystery and evil are almost synonymous." Barbara Ehrenreich looks back with disapproval on the days when breast cancer "went hidden" and attaches sinister meaning to the "invisible radiologist, off in some remote office, who calls the shots and never has the courtesy to show her face with an apology or explanation," as though there could be no good reason for her being somewhere else and needing additional x-rays. Evidently something about the craving for a world without masks—a world where we see face to face, a Rousseauvian world—inspires suspicions of conspiracy. Conspiracy accounts for the darkness and misinterpretation, the trickery and heartlessness that govern a world *with* masks. And corporations, as powerful combinations, make natural conspiracies. Moreover, if the corporations were not responsible for breast cancer, the political thesis of the true believer would not explain everything.

One such ideologue, the author of *Manmade Breast Cancers,* devotes herself to "the theorization . . . of the structural relations of racialized class patriarchal power." Racialized class patriarchal power: epithet follows epithet like a procession of tanks in some May Day parade in the old Soviet Union. After telling how her mother, her mother's sister, two of her own sisters, and she herself were all afflicted with breast cancer, the author proceeds to argue that breast cancer is the product of "a global capitalist patriarchal economy." (I wonder if the same male forces are responsible for prostate cancer.) Owing to a conspiracy of silence, however, the guilt of this vast complex has not been widely recognized. *Manmade Breast Cancers* thus represents itself as an act of "unsilencing."

A friend with breast cancer says, "They never want to talk about causes," by which she means the poisons and pesticides that account, supposedly, for the incidence of cancer in North America. "Cause" is closely linked with "conspiracy"—a conspiracy of greed supported by a conspiracy of silence—and so it was in the eighteenth century. The Enlightenment search for causes translated directly into a widespread suspicion of conspiracy. "When things happen in society, individuals with particular intentions, often called 'designs,' must be at the bottom of them. . . . All enlightened thought of the eighteenth century was structured in such a way that conspiratorial explanations of complex events became normal, necessary, and rational," Gordon Wood writes. Even as the grandchildren of the Enlightenment seek emancipation from the past, they employ a rhetorical style forged 250 years ago. If human beings, endowed with "the capacity to predict and control not only nature but [their] own society," find all going wrong, the explanation must lie in the sinister work of human agents. But in spite of the investment of so many in the theory that breast cancer itself is the work of evil combinations—the corporations responsible for toxins and pollutants—the fact is that "for breast cancer, there is no 'cause' in the straightforward . . . meaning of the word," while some considerable blame for the disease must go to the effects of the body's own hormones on the breast. Such is the complexity of cancer genesis that the very word "cause," as used in cancer debate, is practically an obstacle to clarity.

SO FIXED is the argument that our culture is, or ought to be, advancing from the dark ages of myth to the era of enlightened understanding that a statement like this stands for ten thousand:

> That was back in the Dark Ages, at least in terms of prostate cancer awareness, when even though hundreds of thousands of men developed the disease each year and tens of thousands died from it, prostate cancer was like a big, dark secret.
>
> It's not secret anymore. Today there's a worldwide movement to educate men about the disease. . . .

Proclaiming that we have left the era of ignorance behind, such rhetoric implies that a lot more is known about prostate cancer than is known in fact. Of the available treatments for the disease, including doing nothing, a physician wrote recently in the *New York Times* that "doctors do not know which one is most effective." The literature on prostate cancer is strewn with such confessions of ignorance. Perhaps it was this sort of embarrassment that moved the former director of the Centers for Disease Control to declare,

> It is important that we move toward the development of health messages that reflect the best medical knowledge available to date on prostate cancer to meet the information needs of primary care clinicians and of the public.

Is this anti-language, this speech that withers the human tongue, really better than silence?

On the grounds that so little is known about prostate cancer and so little about its treatment statistically verified, many in the medical world, including the CDC, oppose routine screening for the disease. To me screening makes sense—more sense in some cases than others. But will more men get tested the more they know about incontinence, impotence, even castration? (How calmly, how professionally the doctors write of castration!) Prostate cancer poses a kind of ultimate test of the doctrine that everything can be said and shown. And does anyone really want to make the case that fear of castration, or mere incontinence, is socially constructed—that it is a product of poor social arrangements and in a properly enlightened, "healthy" world would not exist? Even if candor really were a matter of defying prohibitions and inhibitions, I question both the theory that such rhetoric is itself a kind of social medicine and the broad portrayal of the past as a dark age of timidity and silence—even though our forebears lived on closer terms with death than ourselves.

BY AN ODD sequence of events, I once found myself roasting marshmallows by a campfire in a group that included a woman who was once my urologist but had since left the profession. The two of us spoke, and later spoke in private, without the slightest allusion to our history. This was not hypocrisy but the consensual silence of reticence. For their part, Dr. Green and Dr. Marion never asked prying questions, never inquired about anger, concerned themselves with my level of stress, offered psychological tonics of any kind. They too practiced reticence.

With its endless suggestiveness, Brueghel's *Landscape with the Fall of Icarus* is filled with the irony of "saying as little and meaning as much as possible." Also an artist of understatement, Jane Austen kept silent on the issues of the day, an act implying a preference for the traditional institution of literature over its offshoot, journalism. In *Pride and Prejudice,* one scholar has said, nothing and no one of any interest is ever explicit. A page in an Austen novel sometimes reads like a study in elective silence. "Let us have the luxury of silence," says Edmund Bertram to Fanny Price in *Mansfield Park.* Henry Crawford's pressure on her to speak resembles an act of violation. It is because Lady Bertram has no ear for the unspoken that she is a natural dupe for any physician. "With no disposition for alarm and no aptitude at a hint, Lady Bertram was the happiest subject in the world for a little medical imposition." Silence, however, is Fanny's element. "Though never a great talker, [Fanny] was always more inclined to silence when feeling most strongly." Other great novelists endow their characters with fully sexual being without making it explicit (indeed, precisely by not making it explicit). Around their men and women they seem to leave a . . . zone of unexplored freedom, a kind of inviolate spring of independent life. This effect derives . . . from a crucial notion of privacy. There are elements, particularly sexual elements, in their personages which the great novelists fully realize but do not verbalize.

Silence does not necessarily signify a failure of nerve, denial, the repression of the human voice, a conspiracy against truth. "What shall Cordelia speak? Love, and be silent."

Kurosawa once said that before filming a scene he would imagine it played in silence, as in the traditional Noh theater. *Ikiru* (To Live) is Kurosawa's own *Death of Ivan Ilych,* the fable of a bureaucrat leading a false and useless existence until stricken with stomach cancer. (The doctor lies to him, then laughs about it.) On the day after Mr. Watanabe's death, a politician is dishonoring his memory with false speeches when a delegation of women enters and weeps wordlessly at his shrine. A policeman too is shown in silent prayer before the hero's likeness. In a flashback, Mr. Watanabe wears down a superior's resistance to building a park not by argument but by hanging his head in silence. He dies in the park itself, some believe as a mute protest against Town Hall. The film's enduring image is simply of the hero's haunted eyes. "Speech reaches into silence."

From Socrates forward, philosophers have always been cultivators of silence,

> have always defined themselves by their opposition to what can be put publicly into words. Philosophy is secretive, whereas rhetoric is full of public exclamation. . . . Philosophy is secretive precisely in respect of what it knows (or what it seeks), as

was Socrates, who made it part of his self-definition . . . that he never spoke in public.

The rhetorical occasion par excellence is the trial. How ironic, then, that Socrates himself should have been tried. In *The Brothers Karamazov* (which has been placed in the tradition of the Socratic dialogue) forensic categories are themselves put on trial and found wanting. The most remembered and cited portion of *The Brothers Karamazov* must be Ivan's double indictment of God, of which the Grand Inquisitor's argument is but the second half. God is arraigned first for permitting cruelty to children, and beyond that for not relieving a childlike human race of its intolerable burden of freedom. To the Grand Inquisitor's thundering accusations Christ answers not a word. In fact, never in *The Brothers Karamazov* are Ivan's charges against God answered point for point, as though forensically, for in Dostoevsky people do not "argue over *separate points,* but always over *whole points of view.*" That every last point *is* argued over in the trial of Dmitri Karamazov marks that contest a pseudo-event. Precisely as a show that attracts the attention of all of Russia—a public sensation and a stage for rhetorical display— the trial simply does not lend itself to the discovery of a complex truth. Accordingly, the truth flows right through it without being caught, like water through a net. Dmitri did not kill his father, though his actions certainly meshed with those of the murderer. In point of fact the murder could not have been committed without some part being played, by act or omission, by each of the brothers; yet never do they plot out their roles. Only once, briefly, do they even appear in the same scene together. In effect *The Brothers Karamazov* dismantles that pet construct of the Enlightenment, the conspiracy.

In the old days, it is pointed out, the press kept silent about presidential philandering, and cameras did not show Franklin Roosevelt's stricken legs. But even today we instinctively honor the conventions of silence. In the weeks after the destruction of the World Trade Center, when Mayor Giuliani rose to national prominence as leader of the war-scarred city, the press knew better than to dwell on the man's recent prostate cancer. Everyone understood this was not the moment for such talk. "A time to keep silence, and a time to speak." Specially moving was the image of Giuliani alongside the well-loved manager of the Yankees—Joe Torre, another prostate cancer patient—during the World Series of that fall. What was moving was that prostate cancer was not mentioned. As cynical as it generally is, the press was rediscovering the practice of reticence. Nevertheless a pair of researchers undertook to analyze changing patterns in Giuliani's use of pronouns and articles as an index to his inner state. Reporting on this investigation after the mayor left office, a journalist wrote that as a result of prostate cancer, Giuliani seems "to have morphed into a humbler, gentler guy." Silence can be richer, more expressive, even more informative than speech itself.

The unsaid qualifies the said. Even in Homer, renowned for leaving nothing unexpressed, we find tacit speech. When the Phaeacian princess Nausicaa advises Odysseus not to be seen with her in the city lest scandalous tongues exclaim, "Surely he is to be her husband," she puts in the mouths of others a marriage she herself cannot speak of directly, at least not to Odysseus. Odysseus seems to hear what she doesn't say. When the king of the Phaeacians reproaches his daughter for not escorting him to the palace, Odysseus covers her with a lie she alone recognizes, as though completing the exchange of unvoiced meanings. The sexual life of Odysseus—the fullest character in ancient literature—is richly indicated but not portrayed by Homer. Even in Joyce's *Ulysses* there are a lot more sexual thoughts than acts, the most sexually drenched portion of the novel being the record of Molly Bloom's unvoiced speech.

Silence is the depth dimension of speech. *Ulysses* resounds not just with the *Odyssey* but with *Hamlet,* and the whole of *Hamlet* resounds with the untold. "I could a tale unfold." "O, I could tell you— / But let it be." In life, too, not all lends itself to speech. The last clause of the Hippocratic oath binds the physician "that whatever you shall see and hear of the lives of men which is not fitting to be spoken, you will keep inviolably secret."

SELF AND OTHERS

POLLS SHOWING that 90 percent of respondents would like to be told they are dying bring to mind elections where 99 percent vote for the anointed candidate. Why would people imagine they are supposed to report themselves ready and willing to confront death, almost like the titans of Ivan Karamazov's imagination who "accept death proudly and serenely like a god"? Everyone of course thinks courage better than cowardice, and it is; but perhaps, too, as moderns with a belief in reason we feel we should be able to face the facts without blinking, almost as a doctor might contemplate the condition of another. For my part I don't care to know as much as the physicians about some of the stages of prostate cancer. More than once I was stunned with unasked-for stories about patients further along in the disease. Those who leave things to the doctor once seemed to me misguided souls who take their own body for a car you leave with a mechanic. But maybe there are things best not troubled about. Had I insisted on knowing everything, I would also have insisted on remaining awake through surgery, as a recent patient in fact had done. The idea that I should be able to contemplate my own condition clinically, and that not to do so was to fail some obscure obligation to myself, was poorly thought out. I must have absorbed it somehow.

In tracing modern practices of detachment back to their sources in the revolution in thought initiated by, among others, John Locke—himself a physician—the philosopher Charles Taylor underlines the requirement that we separate ourselves not only from traditions and inherited beliefs but, still more radically, from our own selves. Writes Taylor, the philosophy of Locke is informed by the new

> ideal of a human agent who is able to remake himself by methodical and disciplined action. What this calls for is the ability to take an instrumental stance to one's given properties, desires, inclinations, tendencies, habits of thought and feeling, so that they can be *worked on,* doing away with some and strengthening others, until one meets the desired specifications.

One of the standard-bearers of modern culture, this figure shows up today in the person who goes into therapy to work on his problem—the Lockean philosophy itself has been compared to a course of therapy—or the patient working to manage cancer by reconstructing his thinking and habits, or indeed anyone who follows some regimen of self-improvement. Earlier incarnations include James Gatz, later Gatsby, follower of a daily program of self-improvement; and, in history, the thoroughly Lockean Benjamin Franklin, whose scheme to make good use of every hour in the day, to better himself by methodical and disciplined action, is detailed in his autobiography. (In the resolve of cancer patients to "make the most of every day," the voice of Benjamin Franklin is heard at a distance.) To engineer yourself is a solitary transaction. With counsel like "Identify your emotions" and "Live one day at a time," cancer literature sometimes seems addressed to one dropped onto earth from another world, a solitary indeed, a newcomer to human experience without sense, without companions, without a past, simply unacquainted with human ways and the human record, as though history itself had been reduced to a blank slate. An anti-cancer cookbook intended "to help you enjoy the pleasure of food" seems addressed to someone unfamiliar with the practice of eating.

The Job's comforters of cancer insinuate that you brought on the disease by stress. Someone with prostate cancer also begins to receive advice about vitamins and diet. To those who believe it lies in our power to remake our selves and our physical selves—even if, logically speaking, that isn't so different from picking oneself up by the hair—the notion of preventing or even curing illness through some sort of behavioral regimen recommends itself very readily. Imagine a cancer patient set on reconstructing himself from the inside out, dividing the day as follows:

6–7 A.M.	Jogging
7–8 A.M.	Anti-cancer breakfast
8–9 A.M.	Meditation
9–10 A.M.	Massage
10–12 NOON	Yoga
12–1 P.M.	Anti-cancer lunch
1–3 P.M.	Support group
3–5 P.M.	Exercise
5–6 P.M.	Rest
6–7:30 P.M.	Anti-cancer dinner
7:30–8:30 P.M.	Visualization of disease
8:30–10:00 P.M.	Journal and inspirational reading

Ludicrous, but not that much more so than some of the prescriptions in the literature. While to a culture with contempt for the past the project of self-engineering seems novel, my guess is that it appeals so deeply just because it is so deeply ingrained in what Charles Taylor calls the modern identity, whose roots reach back several centuries. Benjamin Franklin himself at about the age of sixteen became a vegetarian, seeking and finding the "greater Clearness of Head and quicker Apprehension which usually attend Temperance in Eating and Drinking." (It was at this time, Franklin records, that he read "Locke on Human Understanding." It was Locke's belief that parents misled by the traditions of bad eating introduce children to an excessively meaty diet.) The Japanese may eat a soy-rich diet, and meditation may have medical value in Indian traditions, but to eat a soy-rich diet and engage in meditation strictly as a way to beat cancer—to meet desired specifications—is a distinctly Western practice. If the construction and reconstruction of the self weren't so much a concern of our own culture, maybe seekers wouldn't be looking to other cultures for tools and materials in the first place.

The same ideal of disengagement that prompts us to experiment with diet, and otherwise work on our own habits and program our own patterns, also bids us confront the prospect of death with detachment and clarity of mind, almost as if it were someone else's end we had in view. I find this ethic of disengagement narrow and impoverished. Like the practice of communing with your own disease hour by hour, the ideal of autonomy governing the modern project of self-mastery comes too close to reducing moral life to a transaction between me and myself. (Some reduce cancer itself to such a transaction, implying that the cause of the disease lies in some defect and its cure in the repair of the self.) Seemingly in defiance of its own title, the handbook *Prostate Cancer: What Every Man—and His Family—Needs to Know* advises the patient that "the time will arrive when you, and you alone, must decide" on a course of treatment. I did not make such decisions alone. In the same pages we learn of a retired air force officer with prostate cancer who asks his son, a physician, for advice. The son refuses, though when the father decides for surgery he says, "Dad, you made the right decision—right for you." Was the son's refusal an act of humility or an evasive maneuver by one seeking to be held blameless?

As he approaches the end, Ivan Ilych is hindered from completing his own death "by his conviction that his life had been a good one. That very justification of his life held him fast and prevented his moving forward, and it caused him the most torment of all." Only when Ivan Ilych abandons the defense of his life and his way of life can he release both his family and himself from suffering. The release of one is the release of the other.

> He was sorry for them, he must act so as not to hurt them; release them and free himself from sufferings. "How good and how simple!" he thought.

In this, Ivan Ilych's last act, it is as though he rediscovers the wife he has detested, the daughter he has ignored, the son who already looks like him when he studied law. As I underwent my own lesser ordeal, from waiting for biopsy results to recovering from surgery, I became keenly aware of my importance to others and theirs to me—and came to understand that these two relations are in fact one.

SOMETIMES I wonder how members of the eighteenth-century culture of sociability could reconcile their social practices with the stoicism so highly spoken of in their age. But the stoic is no cave dweller, and the reduction of passion is itself an element of social practice. As Hume says, even the stoic "feels strongly the charm of the social affections." (In his moving account of Hume's own last illness, Adam Smith reports that his social disposition never left him. "His cheerfulness was so great, and his conversation and amusements run so much in their usual strain, that, notwithstanding all bad symptoms, many people could not believe he was dying." Hume, however, assured the doctor "I am dying as fast as my enemies, if I have any, could wish, and as easily and cheerfully as my best friends could desire.") In my case a kind of restraint was called forth by social affections in the first place. With nothing to do but wait for test results—and once, before taking my business to Dr. Green, this went on for weeks; long enough for a good half-dozen random calls from a windshield repair service—you take care not to make others more edgy than they already are. So it was throughout treatment.

With each biopsy both children were informed so that in case of the worst the news should not catch them unaware. When the third came back positive, my son asked, "Are you afraid?" I thought about it. "Concerned." One thing I was concerned to do was to offer an example for his sake in case he ever confronted the same circumstance. Soon I was to learn that my son, *as* my son, stands double the average risk of prostate cancer. I felt that fact before I knew it, and in seeking to present an example of one more or less at peace, I found a measure of peace in the belief that I might be helping him.

I thought it important, too, not to alarm my parents unduly, especially as they have already survived one child. There is a Chekhov story about a disconsolate cabdriver who has just buried his grown son. Death should have come for him, he feels, but instead "came in the wrong door." I did not want to inflict this kind of grief.

So too, I was determined not to distress my companion, my wife, if I could help it. More than any other, it was this resolve that strengthened me. In one instance it was a thought for my wife that got me literally off my back.

In Brueghel's painting, the sheep graze as they always do. Following my surgery, while I was in recovery, there came a time when Lizzie simply had to go home and let the dog out. At that point I was still on my back and in some dread of getting up, though in order to be discharged I had to do so—and not only that, had to satisfy the hospital that I wasn't about to go home only to race back to the emergency room. All at once the thought crossed my mind that I would surprise Lizzie by being ready to leave when she returned. She had had enough of the hospital for one day, for sure. The next minutes were memorable in an adverse way, but when Lizzie arrived I was ready to go. At some point I would have gathered up the resolve to get on my feet in any event, but the thought of springing a surprise quickened me and put my will into what had to be done.

Some believe that instead of doing the conventional thing—living by the book—Ivan Ilych should have done whatever his heart desired. One day a friend with cancer said, "Life is short. Do what you really want to. Take your clothes off and run naked." I had no wish to run naked. Not only do I not feel that in order to be my real self I need to cast off social trappings and attachments to others, but it was these bonds that kept me moored. According to a certain way of thinking, our relations to others are indeed purely artificial—a "role" that we "play"—and by surrendering to such conventions we betray our true self. Some appear to see cancer as our being's way of avenging this violation. As we read in a book on cancer cowritten by a physician,

> if we play prescribed social roles instead of taking our journeys, we feel numb; we experience a sense of alienation, a void, an emptiness inside. People who are discouraged from slaying dragons internalize the urge and slay themselves.

I confess I find the language of role-playing hollow and alien itself. I am a husband, I do not play at being a husband; a father and not a pretend-father. What if I had not had the benefit of such ties, had been under no obligation to keep composure for others' sake? Prostate cancer is so inscrutable, and carries with it the risk of such wretched if also ridiculous side effects, that it would be easy just to sink into continual worry. The patient has plenty of time to get caught in this vortex, too. From biopsy to report and beyond, there is much waiting; and waiting attracts worry like a vacuum. At the end of her study of totalitarianism, Hannah Arendt reflects on "the redeeming grace of companionship," its power to save the solitary from the "duality and equivocality and doubt" they might otherwise fall into. Likewise in my case: it was others who kept me from succumbing to anxiety and bewilderment.

Not that this possibility has been completely dispelled. Like any other cancer patient, I will need testing for the rest of my life; for the urologist and me, it is till death do us part. Going through the trials of waiting—like the hero of the old romance *Sir Gawain and the Green Knight,* given a full solar year to contemplate his own beheading—I will draw on whatever reserves of patience have been built up over the last months.

IF THERE IS one journey we are destined to make alone like Gawain, it is the journey to death. Yet while each of us must die for ourselves, we do not die by ourselves, necessarily. Donne's "Valediction: Forbidding Mourning" begins:

> As virtuous men pass mildly away,
>   And whisper to their souls to go,
> Whilst some of their sad friends do say
>   The breath goes now, and some say, No;
>
> So let us melt, and make no noise.

Posed simply for purposes of comparison, the image of a man expiring in the company of friends represents a sort of tacit or assumed norm of a good death. Even the allegorical hero Everyman, deserted by one false good after another on the way to death (more or less like Ivan Ilych), doesn't die absolutely alone: his Good Deeds go to the grave with him. In Boccaccio's account of the effects of the plague on the city of Florence in 1348, so great is the violence done to the fabric of life that family members desert their dying. In *The Brothers Karamazov,* the tale of a family's destruction, the agent of the Karamazovs' ruin dies alone, by his own hand.

But it is Ivan Karamazov, a freethinker with only the most tenuous human attachments, whose imagination seems consumed by solitude. (He dreams of remaking the human race like a single self.) By placing Ivan in dialogue with his own doubles, thus making of him a terrible study of duality, the author baffles the very distinction between self and other. In the story of Ivan's knowing, but not altogether knowing, complicity in the murder of his father, Dostoevsky also baffles the Lockean dictum that responsibility extends only as far as consciousness. According to Locke, it would be wrong "to punish one twin for what his twin-brother did, whereof he knew nothing," the innocent brother bearing no responsibility for, because not conscious of, the other's doings. The dealings between Ivan and his "twin" or double, Smerdyakov, yield a different reading. Ivan *is* responsible in some degree for the murder Smerdyakov committed, not because his mind traveled in Smerdyakov's body and not because he knew with clear and distinct, or Lockean, knowledge that he was entering into a compact with Smerdyakov at the time of their fateful conversation earlier in the novel, but because he more or less knew—knew imperfectly but well enough. To Locke's rule that responsibility requires consciousness, Dostoevsky adds an appreciation of the paradoxical quality of consciousness itself. It is as though in his last novel he returned to the foundation of the modern psychological construct in order to *re*construct the principle of responsibility. In the sheer urgency of his interest in responsibility is something that puts Dostoevsky at odds with the therapeutic culture of today, which increasingly supplies the terms of discussion of what were once moral issues.

COMPASSION

THE MODERN PROGRAM of constructing or reconstructing the self lays great stress on my dealings with myself. Some would say that even compassion is such an act.

According to the model of sympathy laid out by Adam Smith in the *Theory of Moral Sentiments,* in feeling for you I really feel for myself. I feel what I imagine I would feel if I were in your position. Never can I really leave my own skin.

> As we have no immediate experience of what other men feel, we can form no idea of the manner in which they are affected, but by conceiving what we ourselves should feel in the like situation. Though our brother is upon the rack, as long as we ourselves are at our ease, our senses will never inform us of what he suffers. . . . By the imagination we place ourselves in his situation, we conceive ourselves enduring all the same torments, we enter as it were into his body, and become in some measure the same person with him, and thence form some idea of his sensations. . . . His agonies, when they are thus brought home to ourselves, when we have thus adopted and made them our own, begin at last to affect us, and we then tremble and shudder at the thought of what he feels.

"At last": it is as though the seemingly immediate and intuitive response of sympathy were really patiently constructed.

No one would deny that Adam Smith's model has some force. During one especially bad biopsy, I found myself telling the doctor in my head, "Have you been through this yourself? I bet not. I bet you have no idea." At such a moment I was an instinctive Smithian. But while Adam Smith's model certainly holds good in some cases, it does not account for the full range of compassion. Here, then, are a number of cases, some fictional, some drawn from experience, that fall outside its purview.

1. In his last moments Ivan Ilych is overcome with a pity that nothing in the tale to this point anticipates or prepares for—that breaks the script he lived by:

> He felt that someone was kissing his hand. He opened his eyes, looked at his son, and felt sorry for him. His wife came up to him and he glanced at her. She was gazing at him open-mouthed, with undried tears on her nose and cheek and a despairing look on her face. He felt sorry for her too. . . .

> Suddenly it grew clear to him that what had been oppressing him and would not leave him was all dropping away at once from two sides, from ten sides, from all sides. He was sorry for them, he must act so as not to hurt them: release them and free himself from these sufferings. "How good and how simple!" he thought.

Surely Tolstoy doesn't mean that Ivan Ilych feels what he imagines he would feel if he were his wife or his son. That is at once too speculative and too roundabout for an action here both depicted and described as simple. By no means is Ivan Ilych as selfbound as the

Smithian model implies. He looks at his son and pities him. He looks at his wife—the wife he has loathed and detested—and pities her. According to the Smithian model, pity "at last" takes effect when we imagine ourselves into the position of another. The final moments of Ivan Ilych simply do not allow, as it were, for an operation that circuitous. If imagination tells us what we would feel in another's position, in this case there is no "would," nothing conditional or supposed, nothing simulated, about the response of pity. Ivan Ilych responds to what his wife and son do feel, not what he himself would feel. What they feel is written on their faces. If it had been a matter of supposition, Ivan Ilych might have supposed his wife was feigning grief as she usually feigns. The fact is otherwise.

2. In a subplot of *The Brothers Karamazov,* Alyosha becomes acquainted with a stricken family consisting of an ex-captain broken by failure, his imbecile wife, a hunchback daughter, a daughter who can't bear the father's buffoonery, and, at the center of the drama, a beloved son dying as a result of a stoning he suffered in the father's defense. The sheer extremity of all this pathos places the classical model of sympathy under a stress it cannot bear. Alyosha feels keenly for the boy Ilyusha, notwithstanding that as the abandoned son of a debauched father he, Alyosha, knows nothing of the boy's fierce love of his father; and he feels keenly for the ex-captain, also without being able to project from his own experience. (The ex-captain is a timorous man who resents his own timidity, while Alyosha is said to be naturally "bold and courageous.") Had Alyosha, confronting this scene of suffering, felt only what he himself would feel under like circumstances, probably he would be simply baffled, for he has never known anything similar; in fact, so extreme are the circumstances of the family that we are hard put to imagine anything sim-

ilar. At one point in the process of coming to know the humiliated captain, Alyosha does get caught up in his own imaginings, overlooking the reality of the captain's position as a man reduced to servility. And in doing this he errs.

3. In a remarkable and cunning tale by Herman Melville of a captain lost in his own imaginings, the Smithian model of sympathy becomes itself a source of error. According to Adam Smith, I cannot tell what another feels except by imagining what I myself would feel under those conditions. In "Benito Cereno," a sympathetic American comes to the aid of a Spanish ship in distress, whose cargo of slaves—unbeknownst to the American—have risen up, killed most of the whites aboard, terrorized the captain, and taken the vessel. For three-quarters of this tale the mind of the American wanders in a maze of supposition, bound in a waking dream, deceived by the charade enacted on the *San Dominick*. At one point, when the Spanish captain mentions with emotion the death of the slaves' owner, the American seizes the sentimental opportunity and imagines himself into the other's position.

> "Pardon me . . . but I think that, by a sympathetic experience, I conjecture, Don Benito, what it is that gives the keener edge to your grief. It was once my hard fortune to lose, at sea, a dear friend, my own brother. . . . Assured of the welfare of his spirit, its departure I could have borne like a man; but that honest eye, that honest hand—both of which had so often met mine—and that warm heart; all, all—like scraps to the dogs— to throw all to the sharks! It was then I vowed never to have for fellow-voyager a man I loved, unless, unbeknown to him, I had provided every requisite, in case of a fatality, for embalming his mortal part for interment on shore. Were your

friend's remains now on board this ship, Don Benito, not thus strangely would the mention of his name affect you."

(As Wordsworth says, "My fancy has pierced to his heart.") The remains are in fact on board. As we learn later, the owner was murdered and his skeleton "preserved" to strike terror into the surviving whites. Trapped in the circularity of his sympathy, imagining the other's case like his own, the benevolent American becomes a study in delusion.

4. With my PSA well into the red zone, my physicians were careful not to overplay the alarm. They were considerate in other ways as well, assuaging fears before I necessarily knew I had them. But because, as physicians, their acquaintance with cancer was quite different from mine, they could not have performed these sympathetic services by asking what they would have felt in my condition. Had Dr. Green been struck with prostate cancer, he would have brought to the disease a fund of knowledge I did not possess, and by virtue of his medical experience might have feared some things more and some less than I did. But that is irrelevant, because he concerned himself with my situation and not with some imaginary version of his own.

A good doctor, open to learning and experience and (unlike Melville's American) skilled in reasoning from case to case, may know what I am going through not only by the simple act of attending but by carrying over things learned from other patients. Said Dr. Marion at one point: "I know. It feels like you're sitting on an egg." And this statement was as welcome as if it had come from the heart. Dr. Marion did not know that I felt like I was sitting on an egg by asking herself what she would have felt in my circumstances.

5. Dr. Green, similarly, had said that on coming out of anesthesia I would feel an intense local inflammation. My first memory, upon awakening, is of his voice—unassuming yet assured—and of just such a sensation as he described, an inflammation unlike anything I had known before. Dr. Green had so prepared me that this strange and overpowering experience, instead of causing panic, actually gave me my bearings. "It's just as he said!"

6. What better proof that compassion does not necessarily flow from a mental change of places than a man's compassion for a woman in labor? By no means can the man imagine himself giving birth, and yet this impossibility does not stand in the way of a strong identification with the woman's suffering, a compassion that flows through the body itself.

7. More subtle was the compassion of my nurses. Without knowing in detail what I was experiencing, and presumably without asking what they themselves would feel as men with radioactive titanium pellets embedded in them, somehow—in the subtlety of their hearts—they understood my position and its sometimes painful absurdity.

HISTORY'S CHILDREN

ON BEING DISCHARGED from the hospital some hours after surgery, I was handed a kit containing guidelines on radiation safety, a steel casing the size of a bullet to store any vagrant seeds in, and plastic tweezers. Also in the kit were packets of condoms along with printed advice on their use "for aesthetic or hygienic reasons." Whenever the physicians brought up the matter of sex, it was in the same spirit: sex, however you practice it, is a normal function. Though they left it at that, I could not help hearing in the easy way these modernists—especially Dr. Marion—had with sex, a judgment on the past: an implied condemnation of the dark ages when the subject was still charged with secrecy. The old practices of repression, they seemed to say, are best forgotten or, if remembered, held up as an example of ignorance like the use of leeches in medicine. At one time physicians warned against masturbation. Now "more frequent masturbation" was advised, on hospital letterhead, as the remedy for side effects of surgery.

Many seem to believe that just as sex itself is natural, so people left to themselves will naturally come to consider it a function and not a mystery. On this showing, the corporation that supplies condoms, the hospital that advises sexual exercise as a health measure, the physicians themselves are all children of nature. I believe, on the contrary, that only after a long campaign of repetition and only because certain ideas have been established over time could a clinical understanding of sexuality seem natural in the first place. In other words, if we weren't so much in history's debt, never could we tell ourselves that history itself is a tale told by an idiot and that we alone understand sex as it really is, without artifice, mystery, or repression.

As I have argued, the liberation rhetoric heard today in the cancer world replays the rhetoric of civil rights introduced a generation ago, with patients now breaking through the inhibitions of shame and traditions of ignorance and oppression. In the name and pose of daring, the users of such rhetoric recite phrases that have already been completely institutionalized. In the same way, if not for a century-long campaign associating the airing of sex in all of its aspects with all that is progressive, emancipated, and medically enlightened, perhaps the virtues of saying all couldn't be taken for granted today. But the campaigners for freedom of sexual discussion did more than throw open a curtain and let the light in. They also blackened the opposition as cowards, hypocrites, and enemies of enlightenment. Hence, for example, the fixed stereotype of the puritan who wreaks his own repression on the world, an uncouth "busybody who will stop at nothing, not even censorship and imprisonment, to impose his self-righteous morality upon others." Even in using the rhetoric of boldness, the party of disclosure played on the fear of being derided as repressed or retrograde, and it may be that even today some people adopt sexual opinions out of the sheer dread of not adopting them, more or less as Ivan Ilych followed the political fashion and became a new man because he was not one to be out of step with prevailing opinion.

BELIEF AND DISBELIEF

IT WAS Montaigne's view that illnesses "have their life and their limits. . . . Anyone who makes an assay at imperiously shortening them by interrupting their course prolongs them and makes them breed, irritating them instead of quietening them down." Nature mocks us, punishing our attempts to cheat her power. Given the state of medical knowledge in his time, Montaigne's disbelief in medicine makes sense. Skepticism as practiced by Montaigne is the art of disbelieving without disbelief becoming a credulity in its own right. By contrast, the conspiracy theorist subjects the accepted version of things to a withering disbelief only to offer in its place a fiction that defies belief. Like those who maintain that the Israelis masterminded the destruction of the World Trade Center, or indeed that the gas chambers never existed, the conspiracy theorist joins a great cynicism to a great credulity. As Hannah Arendt once said of the citizen of the totalitarian state, he believes nothing and believes everything. It is as if he lacked a sense of the probable. Without the guidance of judgment, which enables us to evaluate probabilities informed by our experience of things, we too might be condemned to these mood swings of belief, these ideological chills and fevers. A cancer patient learns very soon the importance of questioning, but also learns that suspicion can go too far. For it just cannot be true that "beneath the appearance of *every* human phenomenon there lies concealed a discrepant actuality," no matter how "firmly entrenched" this doctrine may be. For one who believes that, suspicion has become an idol and penetration a pretense.

As I recall, the mother of a high school friend took Krebiozen, a mineral oil said to be effective against cancer but (we were given to understand) illegal in the United States. Like cancer itself, Krebiozen was something disgusting, mysterious, and remote. That our government would ban a cancer remedy didn't make sense, but neither did other things adults did. If Krebiozen was blacklisted, did not many good people in the McCarthy days receive the same treatment? It never occurred to us that this elixir might have been blacklisted because it did nothing but prey on delusion. The theory that the government is actually committed to suppressing the cure for cancer has a certain vitality to this day in American folk culture.

Perhaps it is the stealthiness of cancer itself that induces the belief that forces of stealth are at work in the world, spreading the disease and blocking its cure. A recent full-page ad in the *New Republic,* a magazine that prides itself on a robust skepticism, bears the title "Black Listed Cancer Treatment Could Save Your Life" and reads in part:

> As unbelievable as it seems the key to stopping many cancers has been around for over 30 years. Yet it has been banned. And kept out of your medicine cabinet by the very agency designed to protect your health—the FDA.
>
> In 1966, the senior oncologist at St. Vincent's Hospital in New York rocked the medical world when he developed a serum

that **"shrank cancer tumors in 45 minutes!"** 90 minutes later they were gone. . . . Time and again this life saving treatment worked miracles, but the FDA ignored the research and hope he brought and shut him down.

You read that right. He was not only shut down—but also forced out of the country. . . .

By simply eating a combination of two natural and delicious foods (found on page 134) not only can cancer be prevented—but in case after case it was actually healed!

In order to believe this traveler's tale you have to regard the FDA as a conspiracy against truth and health, or perhaps be in a state of despair that overwhelms questions of belief and disbelief altogether. The theory that cancer flows from the Cancer Industrial Complex, while more intellectual, is not that different, the wrongdoer in this case too engaging in elaborate exercises designed to convince the world of its benevolence and reduce people to dupes. Back in high school we used to laugh at the notion that the Communists were infiltrating our bodies with fluoride and our minds with propaganda; we did not realize that the left could employ the same rhetoric, this time with the corporations smuggling carcinogens into everyone's bodies and controlling minds by inducing political narcosis.

In the 1980s there appeared in the *New Yorker* an investigation of the dangers of asbestos and what the industry knew or should have known about them. Impressed by the author's research, I attended a lecture by him and took up his next book disposed in his favor—not knowing at the time that he imagines himself "a kind of literary entomologist—one who overturns rocks in the dank garden of the private enterprise system . . . and describes what he sees crawling out from underneath," so committed is he to the principle that under appearances lies a disgraceful reality. In the later book the case is made that emissions from power lines are causing cancer throughout the United States. Not content with probing a single industry, and sailing clear past other exponents of the social theory of disease, the author contended that cancer was literally built into our way of life. He soared high and his wings melted. To the question, "What cause of cancer is everywhere but goes unnoticed?" he offered a reply that was good as answers to riddles go—"electromagnetic fields"—but weak as science. Maybe there is just something irresistibly ironic in the notion that things so taken for granted as power lines should be so dangerous. The same considerations recommend the theory that Coca-Cola leads to bladder cancer. Just as Rousseau's belief that disease is rooted in our way of life almost requires a conspiracy to account for public ignorance of a cause so glaringly obvious, so the power-line theory was promoted as the exposé of a great cover-up. For a while the power-line theory had some play, but any remaining believers must account for the fact that it now goes unnoticed itself; and so another theory is born.

Many theorize that prostate cancer too springs from our way of life—specifically our way of eating, "the Western diet." By the time a man starts thinking about his prostate, habits of diet have been in place for decades, but, like an ideal theory, the Western diet theory nevertheless implies that it is not too late to change. In other words, the effects of the Western diet are at once grave and reversible.

The Western diet theory sounds better than it really is. In a nation with 125 million men you would think such an all-present menace as the Western diet would account for more than 40,000 deaths per year from prostate cancer. If the Western diet really were incompatible with the human prostate, as one medical commentator surmises, wouldn't the figure be higher? At most, diet contributes to prostate cancer without "causing" it. But why do the claims made against the Western diet sound so good? To think that with some dietary effort we can get clear of a feared disease is highly consoling (consoling enough to make up for the horror of having brought the disease on ourselves to begin with). If we can do something about prostate cancer by eating differently, we are not at its mercy. Then too, a fatty diet has been implicated in heart disease, making the same diet suspect by analogy in the other case. The charge that an unnatural diet is destroying us also picks up the strain of naturalism that runs through our culture. As the literary critic Northrop Frye observed a generation ago, "most of us have been brought up in . . . a half-baked Rousseauism," and the indictment of the Western diet rewords Rousseau's indictment of civilization itself as the great source of disease. Accusations of the Western diet tap into the potent belief that there is something fundamentally injurious about Western and especially American civilization—the sort of belief now pushed hard in the universities—without introducing the more lurid political corollaries of this notion. All of this taken together would be more than enough ideological fuel to power suspicions of the Western diet, but in addition there is the seductive irony that our very affluence should be our demise.

In a sharp-witted work, the singular Albert O. Hirschman traces certain devices of conservative argument back to the age of the French Revolution and examines their usage since that time for the purpose of blocking reform. First among these watchwords of reaction is the "perversity" argument, which holds that unwise political attempts are fulfilled in reverse.

Attempts to reach for liberty will make society sink into slavery, the quest for democracy will produce oligarchy and tyranny, and social welfare programs will create more, rather than less, poverty. *Everything backfires.*

Toward the end of his study, the author concedes that reactionaries aren't the only ones to use such tropes. "Their progressive counterparts are likely to do just as well in this regard," and this is very true. Every time a progressive argues that criminalizing drugs only makes the problem worse, a perversity claim is made, a claim much like those exposed by Hirschman as flashy ploys. But what of the contention that the pharmaceutical companies are killing us, that the consumer society is perishing of its own success, that in the corporations we have created a monster, that our quest for the good life has brought cancer on ourselves and our children? Was there ever a more ambitious application of the perversity thesis? Perhaps the argument that the institution of medicine is itself the downfall of health.

The theory that Western medicine is but another form of domination has some credit in the humanities, but is too wild to have much of a public following. But some sort of belief in exotic therapies is definitely in circulation, as though such methods had a special efficacy precisely because they lie outside the bounds of Western medical practice. Think outside the box. Not long after being diagnosed, I heard a medical acquaintance on the radio interviewing someone about the virtues of vibrational healing, the vibrations being produced by the didgeridoo, the large bamboo or wooden trumpet of the Australian aborigines. Just as the aborigines have been oppressed, so (said the guest) the wisdom of aboriginal healing practices has been unwisely ignored. The former dean of a medical school and one of the hundred members of the Osler Society, the interviewer probably doesn't much believe in the healing effect of musical vibrations, and if he were found to have cancer he would not seek out this exact treatment, but being socially conscious he went along with his guest. There are those who believe that aromatherapy can stimulate the immune system, that with practice you can send love to your immune system, that cancer can be repelled by massage, that prostate cancer is caused by stress and dental fillings. Among the anti-cancer agents exciting interest are turmeric and beer. The newspaper reports a "small but significant study" showing that yoga along with the correct diet "may" help men with prostate cancer. All participants in the study "received supportive counseling." Toward these practices some in the medical world may take the attitude of "Whatever works," like the police using psychics. There are also prostate health boosters on the market that look legitimate and, for someone with the warning signs, are hard to resist. Brueghel's plowman simply follows an ox that seems to know its own way. The cancer patient finds himself, or herself, in a Cretan labyrinth of questionable information.

ICARUS CROSSED a line, but where was it? For its part, the line between the medically valid and the merely faddish is ill-marked if marked at all. The cancer patient hears all kinds of assertions not only about diet but about vitamins, "visualization," stress—some advertised as science. "A few years ago, researchers in California discovered that women with breast cancer who took part in support groups survived significantly longer than women who didn't attend." Much as medicine itself shades off into psychotherapy at the ultraviolet end of the scientific spectrum, so do medical findings give way to ideology and vogue. The gap left by the absence of a cure for cancer will not remain unfilled, and in the end somebody—the patient, along with those he or she trusts—must discriminate between good information and the fashions of desperation. One can only hope the abstention from judgment promoted by the therapeutic culture doesn't translate into an ability to make *these* judgments.

There is brachytherapy and there is psychotherapy, but when psychology enters in, the cancer literature fills with a very mushy sort of science. In a work of this genre cowritten by a medical doctor and a psychologist, the reader is notified that "survival can depend upon discovering the subconscious part of your mind that is somehow sabotaging your efforts to stay alive," as in the case of a patient whose ability to envision the cancer within her "allowed her to transform the dark, decaying part of her into a source of life." Elsewhere in the same book we are told of a patient "raised in a religiously very conservative family" who interprets her cancer as punishment for her sins. "For some people it is preferable to believe that they did something wrong to cause their cancer rather than to believe that it 'just happened.'" It is ideologically proper to reduce guilt to conditioning; but it is also ideologically proper to implicate an unhealthy diet and way of life in cancer. So the same authors who have implied that cancer sometimes just happens also hold up as exemplary the case of one who took cancer as a challenge to correct his bad habits and rebuild his life. "He was able to respond to his diagnosis as a message to live a more wholesome life rather than as a threat." Both cases are constructed to current ideological standards. Both patients have been under the spell of bad influences that block their discovery of their rightful selves. (This must be what Northrop Frye had in mind by half-baked Rousseauism.) It would have been improper and unfashionable to present the case of a woman who brought uterine cancer on herself by her incorrect way of life, or the case of a man sunk in "a toxic lifestyle" whose cancer nevertheless did not result from his way of life but just happened. Because ideology can't be sure at this moment whether stress produces cancer or it is just too foolish to suggest that this is the case, the authors conclude that "the relationship between stress and cancer is complex," citing the example of a woman who is "likely" wrong to attribute her cancer to stress. Like coated pills, these and other life-stories are packaged for the reader and go down easily. The authors label their psychomedical approach to cancer a middle way between the extremes of conventional and alternative medicine.

Scanning the literature on prostate cancer (as various as the speeches at Hyde Park Corner), I noticed a volume cowritten by the same pathologist who reviewed two of my biopsies and raised my Gleason score—that Oz of the prostate spoken of with awe by two of my physicians.* ("He'll have the results back in a couple of days unless he's out lecturing. He lectures everywhere.") In addition to medical information, *Prostate Cancer: What Every Man—and His Family—Needs to Know* offers banal social judgments ("Unfortunately, we live in a society that . . ."), therapeutic pabulum ("It's natural to feel angry about what is happening to you"), and the surmise that meditation may enhance the immune system. Though the book has the endorsement of the American Cancer Society and the seal of medical authority, a critical reader will have to sort out a certain amount of ideological chaff. Like the entourage that travels with the president, much that is not medicine has attached itself to medicine.

---

*The Gleason score is an estimate of a cancer's virulence based on the appearance of biopsied cells.

Michael Milken, whose organization CaP Cure underwrites legitimate research into prostate cancer, believes "there is a common collective thought that if positively used can affect the course of history and events and even one's own health."

But finally there is something baffling about this disease of prostate cancer that can kill you but that many live with for years on end—a disease so companionable that many don't even know they have it. A cancer that can move fast or slow, lie dormant or turn deadly, that can be overtreated or undertreated by the removal of the prostate, that it may or may not be advantageous to know about, seems to have some inhuman trickster presiding over it. The father of one friend died of prostate cancer, the uncle of another has lived in peace with it for fifteen years. Knowing full well the dangers of the disease, some physicians still maintain that not treating it at all may be no worse than the existing treatment options. They contend, furthermore, that we have no solid evidence that any treatment really works. Recently I discovered that my internist's grandfather, himself a pathologist, left his own prostate cancer untreated and died with and not of the disease. Like a child who learns a new word and starts noticing it, or like Dickens's Joe Gargery whose reading extends to J's and O's, I seem to be finding this disease everywhere.

In addition to conflicting numbers, contradictory estimates of urgency, and gaps in the evidence, the bewildered patient runs into many lesser puzzles. According to an article in the *New Yorker,* only 5 percent of patients experience "short-term problems of 'urinary urgency'" following the seed treatment; according to information supplied by the hospital where the procedure was later performed on me, the figure is over 75 percent. My father would send me press releases from Sloan-Kettering trumpeting advances in cancer treatment while another informant warned against Sloan-Kettering altogether. "People die there." A urologist in another state advertises his "nerve-sparing" surgical technique in the local Yellow Pages. A licensed physician using a standard term, yet he plays on hope and fear. When a Texas lawyer waged a campaign against the anti-inflammatory Vioxx at the time I was taking high doses of the drug to control the effects of surgery, I was reminded of the equivalent satiric figure of the lawyer as a master craftsman of greed and player on human misery.

With my first appointment with Dr. Marion, the question of just what to believe grew into an enigma. Before meeting with her I viewed a half-hour video on prostate cancer that mentioned the seed treatment once in passing. Later, after Dr. Marion had explained the procedure itself and each and every one of its side effects in detail and with brio, after she had gotten my signature for the seeds and answered such questions as I could put, she asked me to watch a video on the seed treatment. She did so not because she thought it informative but to see if I agreed it was so much "propaganda." Evidently produced by the manufacturer of the seeds, it showed retirees playing golf and tennis and recited the benefits of seeds, all in the manner of a sales pitch. Another production of this kind has implant surgery taking thirty minutes and patients returning to the tee a day or two later—and the better to bring home the ugliness of the alternative shows surgeons hacking away at a prostate gland. (By contrast, a strategic drape keeps too much of the implant procedure from being shown.) The slipcase of the videocassette pictures a man identified as a "67-year-old ironworker who played both golf and tennis three days after being cured by TheraSeed." What physician would use "cured" like that?

A Standard and Poor's report on Theragenics Corporation,

producer of this videotape and manufacturer of radioactive seeds using palladium 103, notes that

> TheraSeed has been shown in independent clinical studies to offer success rates comparable to or better than those for conventional therapies for the treatment of prostate cancer, while being associated with a reduced incidence of adverse side-effects.

While this is fractionally accurate—more accurate in any case than the claim that the ironworker was cured instantly—no one would look to Standard and Poor's for medical information, and perhaps Dr. Marion placed a corporate advertisement in the same worthless category. (In its estimate of the medical value of TheraSeed, Standard and Poor's simply reproduced the corporation's publicity.) For both Dr. Marion and Dr. Green, medicine is medicine: not miracle-working, not holistic healing, not nutritional theory, but medicine.

The radiation given off by seeds is said to work by damaging fast-dividing cells—cancer cells—while sparing their brethren, like God smiting the Egyptians while passing over the Israelites. But that is too simple. In this case too, it seems, my informed consent originated in ignorance.

> A common premise has been that cancer cells grow more quickly than normal. It isn't necessarily so. Unfortunately, the belief that it was [so] provided the basis for mainstay systemic therapy with drugs and radiation that preferentially kill any rapidly dividing cells. It turns out that some cancer cells in fact divide very slowly—but persistently; dominance by stealth. This is true for prostate cancer.

Maybe it was to get at the slow-dividing cells that my doctors used an iodine isotope with the relatively long half-life of fifty-nine days. Still, I am left wondering about cancer cells lying low. So too, the notion that brachytherapy produces negligible side effects, as compared to other treatments for prostate cancer, has now been disputed in the medical literature. The salvational claims made for seeds turn out to be, as Dr. Marion warned, propaganda. But what I could not understand at the time was why Dr. Marion went out of her way to disclaim, in effect, the very procedure she described with such enthusiasm, and would herself be performing. Like one who believes the multinational corporations cloak their crimes in public relations, Dr. Marion wrote off the seed video as a piece of corporate self-interest even as she prepared me for the implant treatment and set in motion the sequence of events leading up to it.

The modest Dr. Green recommended a radical prostatectomy in spite of its dire side effects and in spite of the doubts of many in the medical world regarding such aggressive treatment of early-stage cancer. Dr. Marion dismissed the glowing claims for seeds. In the operating room the two would work in concert, agreeing on the exact placement of something over a hundred bits of titanium, each the size of a grain of rice.

THE WILL TO TRANSPARENCY:
JEREMY BENTHAM

THE NOTION of reconstructing ourselves by breaking old habits and forming new ones, like the patient breaking himself of his toxic lifestyle, has caught on not because it is such a new idea in its own right but, I believe, precisely because it falls in so well with a program for the reconstruction of knowledge, and of the self, laid down centuries ago. In the same way, the suspicion of concealment that governs the preference for disclosure, including the desire to tear the veil from cancer, is but the latest form taken by the practices of demystification inherited from the Enlightenment. Some years before Sissela Bok's *Lying,* Lionel Trilling cited the already

> firmly entrenched belief that beneath the appearance of every human phenomenon there lies concealed a discrepant actuality and that intellectual, practical and (not least) moral advantage is to be gained by forcibly bringing it to light.

As extreme as it is (*"every"* phenomenon), this belief is firmly entrenched because it has so much history behind it, and notable among history's unmaskers was Jeremy Bentham, a specialist in exposing motives who bequeathed to our own era not only terms and categories but a style of problem-solving. Bentham was possessed by a will to transparency, something I could not help thinking of as I underwent one procedure after another that looked right through me. At times I seemed to be in a sort of Benthamite universe where the drapery of things is torn away and the nakedness of numbers remains. I experienced only too much transparency.

Though he likened himself to a physician and confessed a debt to medicine, Bentham himself made no contribution to that science or art. But he did contribute to a belief in publicity itself as a kind of curative force (what he called an antiseptic influence), and his way of reducing problems to calculations has found an echo in medicine. In weighing costs and benefits, even my own physicians proved descendants of Bentham. So indeed do all those (including cancer activists) who argue that the time has come to break traditions of silence, for according to his godson J. S. Mill that is exactly what Bentham did: in disparaging the British constitution, Bentham said what few had dared to say or even think.

THE VANGUARD of the British middle class in the later eighteenth century sought to reform government, strip away the mysteries and archaisms surrounding the oligarchs of England, and subject fictions to public light. These became Bentham's causes. For decades he campaigned to clear up the English law—a thicket of confusion planted by cunning lawyers—and in the radicalism of old age pressed for measures such as the secret ballot and manhood suffrage that reformers had advocated a generation before. In his critique of the medievalism of the English political system, Bentham argued for the greatest happiness of the greatest number, a standard that seemed to him more rational than the vague pieties usually appealed to in debate. In place of a cosmos ruled by mystery and traced with the signature of higher meanings, he wanted a regime of clarity, which is also to say a regime of law. For in a world of law and not mystery, statutes have a truly public character, speaking "a language familiar to everyone." Though Bentham's prose is notoriously illegible, it was a rage for clarity that moved him to write it. If utilitarianism in one version or another now supplies many of the terms and categories of public discussion, it was Bentham who gave that creed its most public and influential expression.

Anatole Broyard, dying of prostate cancer, wrote that a good doctor would "use his science as a kind of poetic vocabulary instead of using it as a piece of machinery." Bentham equated poetry with a game of push-pin, and to Thomas Carlyle, at least, it seemed that he pictured a human being as a piece of machinery. In a slighting reference to Bentham and his methods of calculation, Carlyle writes that "to fancy [man] a dead Iron-Balance for weighing Pains and Pleasures on, was reserved for this . . . latter era." Bentham, he claims, reduces the living symbol of the universe to a dead mechanism.

In symbols is a "wondrous agency," the wonder being that they reveal and conceal at the same time (much as a parable might veil the very truths it conveys). But this property of the symbol—its power to disclose and withhold a higher truth—suggestively corresponds with the traditional right of those who possess the power of agency in the most wondrous degree to close their councils and intentions to common view while yet displaying themselves in a brilliant and forcible light. Shakespeare's Henry IV tells his son to keep out of the common eye, so that when he does show himself people will be properly dazzled. In the medieval church the same impressive and richly symbolic ceremonies enacted before the people shielded the sacred from them. There was thus "a secret at the inner core of publicity: the latter was based on an *arcanum*; mass and the Bible were read in Latin" rather than the vernacular. During Bentham's formative years such contradictions reached their height in France, where judicial procedures were secret and judicial punishments public (both procedures and punishments became Bentham's obsession), and where the theatrical nature of monarchy itself seemed to many (like the corporations to many today) a cover for corruption.

It is said that in the French Revolution "the order of figuration" was challenged by "the order of representation," image by sign, icon by abstraction, theater by print. In Bentham's ideal world the pomp and rhetoric of power would give way to the simplicity of representation, with pillars and spires becoming more like dots and dashes. Bentham's political writings in particular reflect a will to transparency. Possessed, like the revolutionaries of France, by a drive for transparency, but repelled by the excesses of the Revolution and more intent on checking power than unleashing it, Bentham would have legislators swear to speak on all occasions with "the greatest degree of *transparency,* and thence of simplicity, possible." I imagine Bentham would have approved of a consent form that said, "The details of the operation or procedure have been explained to me in terms that I could understand."

For Bentham there is too much of the traditional theater of power in the symbol, and his animus against the first makes him a critic of the second. Publicity, therefore, is the clearing of mystery and the letting in of light, but without the excesses associated in

France with these drives. Though in his earlier phase he thought of persuading enlightened despots to enact his schemes, Bentham was never a power-worshiper like Carlyle. Traditional power, like a symbol in which "there is concealment and yet revelation," masks its deeper intent even while dramatizing itself. Bentham resented that concealment. He dreamed of a world of glass.

IN THE BEGINNING, according to Rousseau, people "could see into one another's hearts." Through all of its twists, the thought of Rousseau pursues the aim of clearing away whatever now conceals heart from heart. Although the division of labor and the multiplication of wants have corrupted humankind, it is possible, Rousseau imagines, "to regain the transparency we have lost." So great was Rousseau's antipathy to masks that he judged the theater a source of corruption and favored in its place civic games and festivals (of which a rough equivalent today might be the breast-cancer run). While no Rousseau, Bentham too craves transparency. "Why should we hide ourselves if we do not dread being seen?" Bentham was particularly good at tearing away the screens and masks deployed by a corrupt political establishment. Where Rousseau battles "obstruction," Bentham exposes the tactics used to obstruct rational debate. And where Rousseau dreams of moral reformation, Bentham dreams of building reformatories.

Certainly the most colorful of Bentham's schemes for reform is his plan for a human observatory, the Panopticon. Designed so that an inspector could keep inmates under surveillance from a central vantage point, the Panopticon was intended in the first instance for prisons, but also for factories, schools, and any other institution where human beings were to be regulated. As a well-lit facility intended to improve those held within, the Panopticon posed a bizarre variation on such contemporary civic improvements as streetlighting and hospital reform. A hundred years later, when a social worker wrote that the new science of correction

> sentences to a hospital by preference rather than to a dungeon. It sentences to cleanliness, good food, and wholesome discipline, and not to infection and degradation,

he was practically quoting Bentham. For to Bentham, reform in the final analysis meant the reconstruction of human character, an end more effectively promoted, in theory, by the healthful regimen of the asylum than the brutality of the jail. In the interest of health and wholesomeness, inmates of the Panopticon were to be denied beer, tea, and tobacco.

According to Bentham, the Panopticon could actually serve as a hospital. No matter whether your purpose is "punishing the incorrigible, guarding the insane, reforming the vicious, confining the suspected, employing the idle, maintaining the helpless, curing the sick, instructing the willing in any branch of industry, or training the rising race in the path of education," your solution, says Bentham, is the Panopticon. In this claim, which sounds very much like a publicist's exaggeration or an effort to woo sponsors, we detect that confidence in an abstract blueprint—in a "system"—that gave reformers like Bentham a name for naiveté among their opponents. And the abstract perfection of the Panopticon owes something to its shape, based on a circle. The wheel, traditional instrument of torture, gives way to a wheel of cells with an inspector at the hub. Just as Bentham repudiated the traditional cosmos—a world traced with the signs of a higher power—his correctional schemes were meant to supplant the tradition that traced infamy on the bodies of crimi-

nals and attached the most urgent symbolic meaning to the last public gestures of the condemned. Bentham does away with fetters and
torture, and in place of a dungeon proposes a dome of light. His
predecessors are those theorists who sought to civilize not by crude
repression and the threat of damnation but by putting the more innocent passions, like the elementary desire for economic gain, to
enlightened use.

The Panopticon was Bentham's pet project: he promoted the
idea obsessively (at one point securing the approval of William Pitt)
but mostly without results. The harshness of the scheme, however,
has given it fame, and some now see it as the very archetype of
bourgeois society's methods of discipline and surveillance. The influence of the Panopticon is felt even today in the use of one-way
mirrors, surveillance cameras, and electronic eavesdropping, though
Bentham's rage for transparency is also evoked by modern architecture's repudiation of ornament and its aggressive pretense of showing all, its façades of glass. (Bentham's description of the Panopticon
as an "Iron cage glazed" applies more or less to the skyscraper. If a
Panopticon had been built in England, it would have been as archi-
tecturally novel as the skyscrapers in their time.) Today, in discus-
sions of the mechanics of domination, social critics remind us of
Bentham's grotesque ambition of improving people by housing
them in modernistic cages under a warden's all-seeing eye.

BENTHAM'S PRISONERS would walk in wheels for exercise. Otherwise they "would toil for fourteen hours a day, immured in tiny
cells, deprived of the most basic privacy." The denial of privacy is
the most infamous feature of the Panopticon and the mainspring of
its punitive mechanism. For the inspection house is designed so that

at any time the inmates can be observed in their cubicles by the warden at the hub of the structure, himself hidden by the ingenious use of screens. In stark contrast to public buildings like churches, laid out for many to watch a single event, the Panopticon is designed for one to watch many, who are themselves the event. The residents of the Panopticon are subject to constant surveillance; and, most important, they know it.

> The more constantly the persons to be inspected are under the eyes of the persons who should inspect them, the more perfectly will the purpose of the establishment have been attained. . . . The persons to be inspected should always feel themselves as if under inspection, at least as standing a great chance to be so.

Bentham theorized that the sensation of being watched would chill people into behaving themselves, resulting in docile prisoners, efficient workers, or whatnot. If he thought of the Panopticon as a sort of factory that grinds the deviancy out of its inmates, driving that factory is the power of inspection, a moral force seemingly as irresistible as gravity and as elementary as light. The Kantian principle of publicity enjoins you to act in ways "fit to be *seen*"—not only by human observers but by an omniscient God. The inmates of the Panopticon make sure their behavior is fit to pass the inspection of a warden or factory-master who plays God. Placed to see all while remaining hidden, the inspector has the "invisible omnipresence" of a deity, except that godhood is now an illusion of engineering, a piece of trickery, a stage effect.

While promoting the Panopticon as, among other things, a place for curing the sick, Bentham also promised "a new mode of obtaining power of mind over mind."

[115]

Morals reformed—health preserved—industry invigorated—
public burthens lightened—Economy seated, as it were, upon
a rock—the gordian knot of the Poor-Laws not cut, but un-
tied—all by a simple idea in Architecture!

In other words, the Panopticon was Bentham's Modest Proposal, except that where Swift's persona avowed "in the sincerity of my
heart, that I have not the least personal interest in endeavoring to
promote this necessary work," Bentham had the strongest personal
interest in the Panopticon: he was to be the establishment's manager
and foresaw huge profits. In his enthusiasm Bentham even dreamed
of "revolutionizing the world" through the Panopticon, without
introducing the turmoil and "anarchical fallacies" of the French
Revolution. The imperative of transparency that fueled the Revolution—the condition of not having secrets or conspiratorial designs—would be imposed in the Panopticon as a disciplinary
measure. An explosive demand becomes a mechanism of control.
Intended as a "model community subject to the dictates of reason
alone," the Panopticon reads like some French Revolution under a
glass dome. Precisely as a model community it also prefigures the
tourist attraction. Bentham envisioned it as just that, in fact—a place
of wonder open to paying visitors, a kind of Xanadu for profit. The
philosopher of publicity dreamed of making the Panopticon a public attraction. Transformed into an "Aladdin's cave of colour, perfume, and lights," the grounds around the prison would be the
Disneyland of the day.

Throughout his proposals for this prison of his dreams, Bentham takes an I-it stance toward the inmates. They are material for
him to shape, objects for him to manipulate, labor for him to com-
mand, fates for him to dispose. As the prospective manager of the

prison, Bentham writes about his charges with a sense of absolute proprietorship. Claims Alasdair MacIntyre, "It is necessary, if life is to be meaningful, for us to be in possession of ourselves and not merely the creation of other people's projects, intentions, and desires." Bentham, however, conceives the inmates as entirely his— stuff to imprint his purposes on. Balked by the government, he reacts with the indignation of a person swindled out of a treasure rightfully his. The same excess of self that disposed him to think of prisoners as his due in the first place (and more generally led him to think of unfree peoples as his natural constituency, made for his political experiments), also made him magnify a personal humiliation into a national scandal. In his belief that he was the victim of a sinister conspiracy, Bentham was not far behind Rousseau. If the will to transparency leads to melodrama, which in turn assigns "a clear and unambiguously legible meaning" to every event, Bentham believed in clear meanings and took a strictly melodramatic view of the miscarriage of his plans for the Panopticon. Like some worthy commoner in a drama or a cause célèbre, he had been undone by scheming noblemen.

A critic of the Russian intelligentsia was later to observe that the political hero "regards everything around him as material or a passive object on which he can act." As we know, Bentham took exactly this view of his prisoners, and it may be that he felt infamously cheated not only of the profits due him but of the heroic status that would be his as the father of a grand invention. (As Swift might say, whoever could transform prisoners into "sound, useful members of the commonwealth would deserve so well of the public as to have his statue set up for a preserver of the nation.") In any event, one great irony of his invocations of the public good is that few members of the actual public could have shared his belief that the world had been denied a wonderful instrument of improvement. Bentham could let himself think and speak of prisoners as possessions because he was convinced he had their interests and not just his own at heart, even if he meant to work them fourteen hours a day with a state-secured monopoly on their labor.

As to the state itself, Bentham viewed that too with the strictest suspicion. Indeed, he wanted to train the light of observation not only on the underclass—beggars, felons, the unskilled—but on the highest political authorities, placing the former under the eye of the warden, the latter under "the watchful and tutelary eye—the antiseptic influence—of the Public-Opinion Tribunal." (The idealization of publicity as a sort of medical force contributes to the belief of many today that publicity can cure injustice and indeed represents a weapon against cancer.) In other words, Bentham's wish to strip the authorities of their traditional privilege of secrecy and expose them to the check of public criticism was the reverse side of his wish to subject the lower orders to an iron regimen of observation. It is just because Bentham distrusted public officials so much that he proposed to take personal charge of the Panopticon and its residents. In the Panopticon "there ought not anywhere to be a single foot square, on which man or boy shall be able to plant himself—no not for a moment—under any assurance of not being observed," nor can the authorities be permitted any escape from public view and criticism, not even the cover afforded by a rhetorical mask or screen. It is Bentham's desire to deny public officials every last inch of maneuvering room that accounts for the minute, practically paranoid detail of his *Constitutional Code.* As in the Panopticon, the principal check on misconduct is vigilant inspection.

Concerned as he was with the prevention of misconduct and indeed the complete reform of government (as well as with the design of a novel reformatory), Bentham saw himself as a man of benevolence, notwithstanding that his own philosophy pictures human beings as driven by self-interest. In order for institutions to be well designed, someone in this world must have large views and enlightened sympathies, and Bentham presented himself as one such. In effect he placed himself in a different category from ordinary mortals, just as the warden occupies a different category from the inmates by virtue of his vision. If it had ever come into being, Bentham's world would have been one of marked asymmetry, almost as one-sided as the Panopticon, with a few like himself possessing the philosophical vision and the spirit of benevolence so generally lacking in humankind.

WE RESIST making ourselves transparent to others. "We wish to disclose of ourselves no more than we think right and nobody wishes to disclose all of himself," Alasdair McIntyre writes. "We need to remain to some degree *opaque* and *unpredictable,* particularly when threatened with the predictive practices of others." Engineered to deprive people of all opacity and to make them behave predictably, the Panopticon seems to violate human nature itself. But the sort of penetrating inspection so ominous as a mechanism of control (in Bentham's fantasies and blueprints at least) serves beneficial purposes in medicine.

When my third biopsy was reviewed, and the tumor upgraded, by someone represented as the preeminent specialist in the field—a celebrity doctor, in fact, very much like those consulted by Ivan Ilych, some high priest of the prostate—I resented this distant figure I could not see but who had seen the fatal flaw in me. (In time I did get a look at him.) But whatever the arrogance of this authority, word of the regrading of the tumor came from the modest Dr. Green, who himself went on to calculate my chances by consulting a set of tables. From blood tests that yielded maddening results to postoperative x-rays revealing a single seed that had somehow migrated out of place—the sort of chance occurrence that goes into the making of cancer itself—I had to get used to the idea of being an open book for professional eyes to read. "To be so easily seen through I am afraid is pitiful," says one of Jane Austen's heroines. Before surgery a bone scan, an ultrasound volume study, a CT scan, a chest x-ray, an electrocardiogram; after surgery, another chest x-ray, a pelvic x-ray, an unscheduled ultrasound, and another CT scan, the last again reinterpreted by some remote expert unknown and unseen. Under arrest and forced to remove his clothes so that they can be examined by the authorities, Dmitri Karamazov experiences a pang of shame:

> All were clothed, while he was naked, and strange to say, when he was undressed he felt somehow guilty in their presence, and was almost ready to believe himself that he was inferior to them, and that now they had a perfect right to despise him.

Something like that shame ran through my experience, heightened or lowered depending on the moment and, especially, the manner of the others present. Maybe it was the terrible sense of standing exposed that led Anatole Broyard to liken the cancer experience to "moving from a cozy old Dickensian house crammed with antiques, deep sofas, snug corners, and fireplaces to a brand-new one that was all windows, skylights, and tubular furniture"—a house of glass, a Panopticon. Yet my doctors never claimed to be all-seeing or all-knowing. Dr. Green freely admitted his inexperience, Dr. Marion that she did not fully understand how the seeds, once implanted, act on the prostate; and both had the effectiveness of their work (that is, my surgery) reviewed and graded downward by the Seattle Prostate Institute, which found less of the prostate irradiated than they thought. And for all the inspections, some of them really violating, I never had any cause to feel like a captive in an observatory, for who after all had sought these professionals out?

ALTHOUGH Bentham's visions of a prison as a house of hygiene bring to mind the effort to reform hospitals; although he promoted the Panopticon as a facility for curing the sick and even likened himself to a physician, still his scheme does not really translate into medical terms. Nor is it possible to translate the art of treating a patient into a campaign to treat an entire society.

"The art of legislation," wrote Bentham,

> is but the art of healing practised upon a large scale. It is the common endeavour of both to relieve men from the miseries of life. But the physician relieves them one by one: the legislator [his own imagined identity] by millions at a time.

Particularly for one who despised poetry, this is an extravagant metaphor. You cannot practice medicine on millions at a time. The 103 seeds embedded in my body were made for that purpose alone and would have been unsuitable for anyone else (even assuming a radioactive element, constantly decaying, could be put back on the shelf to wait for another use). They were simply untransferable. So is medicine itself untransferable into any other endeavor. What would happen if the kind of inspections and violations that accompany medical treatment were somehow carried out on a grand scale in the name of a political conception of health? In China women were (are?) x-rayed to make sure of their IUDs; in the Soviet Union dissenters were locked up in psychiatric "hospitals." As much as anything else, it is the principle of transparency that makes the very ideal of utopia chilling, even abhorrent. In More's Utopia there are "no taverns, or alehouses, or brothels; no chances for corruption; no hiding places; no spots for secret meetings. They live in the full view of all." And it is in the utopian tradition that Bentham's Panopticon is rooted.

In another version of the dream of transparency, cancer patients are encouraged to see through the myths that confuse and enthrall them, to deny cancer its hiding places by visualizing it (like the woman who in her mind "actually looked at and transformed the dead part of her"), and to rebuild and renew themselves step by step. Where Bentham saw his dream balked by a conspiracy, counselors of this school tend to cast parents, institutions, traditions as a sort of joint threat to our very selves, a conspiracy to keep us from so much as discovering who we really are. Meanwhile, for all the advances made in decoding it, cancer itself remains somehow inscrutable and opaque in the end, if only because of the role played in the disease by sheer chance. Even if each of us could read our own genetic code like an open book written in dots and dashes, we would still not be in a position to calculate our risk of cancer.

IN HIS *Constitutional Code* Bentham is an architect of bureaucracy. But bureaucracy itself is a prison with many confines, wards, and dungeons. Daily I spend hours in such a complex, a world to be entered only by passing through some sort of warp. In this closed system, amid wheels that turn to no purpose, reality loses its character altogether and becomes simply a belief held in common. Here real-

ity is not something to be acknowledged but worked up and packaged, as though it were the output of a toy factory. Cancer in this
context becomes my own reality, something not to be denied, inar-
guable, kept to myself as a private emblem of defiance—like some
ruby a jewel thief might keep in his pocket as he walks down the
street in full view of the world.

CALCULATION VERSUS
JUDGMENT

MUCH LIKE Bentham exposing the fallacious use of epithets, some argue that the term "impotence" ought to be discarded in favor of the more clinical "erectile dysfunction," thus removing both the shadow of hopelessness and the sting of shame. There is something of Bentham in the prostate literature. A list of the clinical stages of prostate cancer reads like some Benthamite table of classifications. (Apparently it was their logic of classification that drew Bentham to books of medicine in the first place.) In construing a seed video as a reflection of its maker's financial interests, Dr. Marion similarly followed Bentham. To Bentham we are creatures of self-interest, just as his hope for the Panopticon itself was blasted by the self-interest of the powerful.

Dr. Marion seemed a kind of born Benthamite in her approach to medical problems as well. Not that she subordinated the patient's interest to some abstraction called the greatest happiness of the greatest number, and not so much that she made no judgments about how people get their happiness, but simply that she believed the way to work out medical problems was by calculation. *La méth-*

ode numèrique. With her everything was percentages. There was a 3 to 7 percent chance, following surgery, of chronic cystitis. Postpone surgery three months and there would be a 1 percent (which I suppose was her way of saying small) chance of metastasis. After the implant itself, it was determined that 86 percent of the prostate was completely irradiated, a figure later corrected to 82 percent. Believing that human questions could be solved by calculation, Bentham also supposed he had the method of calculation in hand; hence his caricature by Carlyle as one "counting-up and estimating men's motives," "checking and balancing." If I understand Dr. Marion, she played down the state-of-the-art procedure she herself performed because, *being* state of the art, it was too recent to allow reliable calculation of long-term results. (Presumably for this reason, brachytherapy is barely mentioned in some cancer literature.) A real Benthamite, interested in security of expectations, prefers more solid data. Statistical information, it is said, now and then conflicts with a doctor's clinical experience. Sometimes the statistics are vindicated in the end, and sometimes the clinician. The clinician in Dr. Marion was content with seeding while the statistician regarded the procedure as unproven. Being no great statistician myself, I accepted the data showing no higher rate of recurrence after seeding than after removal of the prostate, even though the data goes back, as she said, only ten years. That was good enough. The rest I took on trust, a word absent from the Benthamite vocabulary. Perhaps embarrassed by this traditional sentiment, Dr. Marion could speak with ease and even enthusiasm of male anatomy and sexual function, but never did she speak of trust.

In the case of prostate cancer, a fixation on statistical data may block treatment and even diagnosis, for data of the required quality do not exist. On the basis of a meticulous review of the statistical evidence, the Centers for Disease Control recommend against routine screening for the disease. When the CDC announces on its website that "Every 3 minutes, a man is diagnosed with prostate cancer," it is hard to say whether this is an announcement of an emergency or a criticism of scaremongering and overdiagnosis. It was a statistician opposed to mass screening who argued sardonically, but with an eye to the greatest good of the greatest number, that lives could be saved if all men had their prostates and all women their breasts removed at age fifty; his point being that screening comes with costs. Like this ironic spirit, some in the medical world question even the radical prostatectomy, the first choice of so many urologists including Dr. Green, on the grounds that its real value is unknown (if only because many cancers of the prostate never come to anything and thus could be left untreated, while in other cases cancer has already escaped the gland itself). Taking a strict view of the data, one could either choose surgery on the grounds that the alternative is unproven, or reject surgery on the grounds that it is of unproven value itself. Troubled with the lack of controlled tests of one treatment against another, some contend that at present no one really knows how to treat prostate cancer or even whether any treatment is better than doing nothing. As noted, some oppose even testing for the disease because so little is known, mathematically speaking, about its treatment. These purists sometimes remind me of the Flying Islanders of *Gulliver's Travels,* so mathematical that they cut their mutton into equilateral triangles.

> Although they are dextrous enough upon a Piece of Paper, in the Management of the Rule, the Pencil, and the Divider, yet in the common Actions and Behaviour of Life, I have not seen a more clumsy, awkward, and unhandy People.

For all their own numerical scruples, the physicians who treated me were dexterous in every respect, a quality well suited to the world of uncertainty in which we have to make our way.

In a departure from their usual good sense, the editors of the *New Republic* pointed out in 1996, to candidate Bob Dole's disadvantage, that "the average 72-year-old white man suffers a 27 percent risk of dying within five years" while for the average forty-nine-year-old white male "the risk is 4 percent." Readers were exhorted to ponder that twenty-three-point difference. Is this bit of socio-actuarial projection a serious political argument or a Swiftian parody? Commenting on the mentality of the "problem-solvers" who planned the Vietnam War, Hannah Arendt might almost have had Swift in mind when she wrote that they "did not *judge*; they calculated. . . . [They] lost their minds because they trusted the calculating powers of their brains at the expense of the mind's capacity for experience and its ability to learn from it." With her portrait of problem-solvers duped by their own love of percentages and their own habit of balancing risks and returns, she could have been describing Swift's proposer, who indeed loses his mind to his calculations and humbly imagines himself a national savior.

Prostate cancer is a city of numbers. Autopsy reveals evidence of prostate cancer in 30 percent of men over fifty. Autopsy also reveals evidence of prostate cancer in a certain percentage of men from thirty to forty-nine. In certain studies, 87 percent of men with lower-grade tumors and 34 percent with higher-grade tumors survived without surgery or radiation for ten years. (In a postoperative visit, I myself was told I would not have lived ten years without treatment, though how Dr. Marion came by this knowledge I have no idea.) Rates of incontinence following surgical removal of the prostate vary, by one source, "from 2 to 59 percent." According to another source, following removal of the prostate, "somewhere between 20 and 90 percent" of men will be impotent. In the grey jargon of medical literature, removal of the prostate "may influence quality-of-life."

Like the International Index of Erectile Function (IIEF), many of these statistics seem like products of some suspended sense of the inane. The numbers confronting the prostate cancer patient mask a good deal of vagueness. In my own case, cancer cells graded 2 on the Gleason scale by one pathologist were graded 3 by another; as I was later told, it is just as if two viewers gave a painting different ratings on their scale of beauty. But if a certain chart is correct, by raising my Gleason score the renowned pathologist moved me from a 6 to 11 percent to an 18 to 30 percent chance of dying within fifteen years. He did that with a stroke of his almighty pen. But when the time came for us to decide on a course of treatment, we couldn't follow the numbers because on one critical point there were no numbers. I don't mean that no statistics exist on the success rate of the seed treatment, but that Dr. Green had performed the operation only once, under supervision, and therefore had no success rate of his own. If someone had asked two or three years ago if I would allow a doctor to learn on me, I would have said Positively No. Experience is a great chastener. I had learned enough about Dr. Green to trust him. As he pointed out, the seed procedure resembles the technique used to biopsy the prostate, and his biopsy technique was meticulous. In fact, so much more careful was his work than his predecessor's—he took more samples, for one thing—that I wonder even now if he simply found what the other missed. That Dr. Green freely admitted his inexperience, with no shuffling, spoke well of him. I asked him if he believed himself competent to perform the seed implant. Again without hesitation, he said yes. That was good enough.

When Dr. Marion dismissed the claims made for a procedure that she herself performed, there was something in her manner of false modesty and something of a strict respect for numbers. When Dr. Green advised removal of the prostate without even mentioning the possibility of a less radical treatment, this was probably because surgery is the likeliest way to get rid of the cancer, but also because he didn't have the immodesty to recommend, in preference to the standard procedure, one he was only beginning to learn. Between his understatements and her flamboyance, the two are yin and yang, she the pride, he the subtlety of human skill. So complementary and so much in accord are these two that they give the illusion that medical disagreement belongs to the days of Ivan Ilych.

In placing trust in Dr. Green, however, we were placing trust in another as well. It was as if circumstances had conspired to underscore the importance of judgment by putting us and keeping us in a position where we had to decide whether or not to trust. As one just learning the procedure of the seed implant, Dr. Green would be performing the operation (in concert with Dr. Marion) under a proctor; and that proctor would be the gentleman I inherited when my original urologist of many years retired—the gentleman I left for Dr. Green. With Dr. Williamson I had a bad history. Owing to reports getting lost inside his office, as well as other sources of delay and acts of indifference, we had to wait at one point three weeks for biopsy results that should have taken a few days, and when word finally did come (not from Dr. Williamson and not from his office) I was on the point of stationing myself in his waiting room and informing the receptionist and anyone else interested that I would not leave without those results in my hands. Some months later, after an alarming blood test, I went to his office and scheduled a biopsy myself. That was what dealing with Dr. Williamson was like. Dr. Williamson took my displeasure very ill and asserted that matters had been handled by his office with all possible efficiency. Dr. Williamson lacks a human touch, his biopsy technique leaves a lot to be wished for, and he shaves his head like someone on Death Row, but nothing suggested that he was so depraved as to avenge himself on me in the operating room or so reckless as to do this in front of three other physicians. I trusted Dr. Williamson.

In an ordinary economic transaction the element of trust is at a minimum. At least things have stated prices. Like any other surgical procedure, a seed implant doesn't conform to this model at all, if only because there is no way to know in advance what complications may arise. (The five seeds they were unable to install weren't billed, it seems.) The doctor-patient relation cannot be reduced to the simplicity of an economic exchange. Insurance helps; but as things unfolded I signed for the seeds before we had authorization from Blue Cross to go forward with the seed treatment at all. Throughout this time, events themselves seemed to be reminding us that even in the era of postmodern medicine, with its CT scans and precise calibrations, its long bills and its perfect indifference, the traditional sentiment of trust cannot be eliminated from human affairs.

Nor of course can all risks be calculated, or should they be. Reflecting that "sexual activity might be causally involved in risk" of prostate cancer, a serious cost-benefit analyst would weigh the gains of such activity against the risks of eventual cancer, as though each episode of pleasure represented the loss of so much of the precious capital of life. Who wants to live by a table of calculations? A man determined to minimize his risk of prostate cancer—it was Bentham who invented the word "minimize"—would have himself preemptively castrated, for eunuchs do not get the disease. Such is the price of secure expectations.

CALCULATION, BIRTH, DEATH

IN A HIGH-SPIRITED mock sermon on trust and distrust, Rabelais—another physician—observes that one who doesn't owe has no one to pray for his long life, while the debtor is surrounded by well-wishers. In a world without lenders and borrowers, Faith, Hope, and Charity would disappear, their places taken by "Mistrust, Contempt, and Rancour." (I can't read this without thinking of Polonius: "Neither a borrower nor a lender be.") On the other hand, a world where everyone lends and everyone owes restores the harmony of the Golden Age. "For Nature has created man for no other purpose but to lend and borrow," in proof whereof Rabelais opens the human body and shows its organs all borrowing from one another.

> Yet this is not all. This borrowing, owing, lending world is so good that when [the] act of feeding is over, it immediately thinks of lending to those who are not yet born, by that loan perpetuating itself, if it can, and multiplying itself by means of its own replicas; that is, children.

In Rabelaisian terms, then, much as the feet trust the hands and both the heart, so do the parents trust to the child for the continuation of their own being. Of course Rabelais doesn't mean to be taken too literally, but perhaps his account of human procreation as an act of trust and hope contains an element of truth missing in modern doctrines of calculation. We millions who were born in the years immediately after World War II—a war the United States emerged from not only undestroyed but stronger than before, and with a new preeminence in the world—are ourselves a testament to hope. But the fact is that no one calculates risks and returns, costs and benefits in having a child. No one has children as a Benthamite. Our very existence on this earth illustrates the limitation of a way of thinking that overrates the importance of calculation in human life.

There is something fitting in the fact that two of history's most famous utilitarians had no children. Bentham never married. When only thirty-one he wrote to his brother, then contemplating leaving England, "O my Sam, my child, the only child I shall ever have, my only friend, my second half, could you bear to part with me?" To John Stuart Mill, Bentham stood as a kind of intellectual godfather. Mill did marry but had no children, though he accepted as his own daughter one not fathered by him, Helen Taylor. His famous essay *On Liberty* adverts to marriages that have "called third parties into existence." One who marries, writes Mill, encourages another to "build expectations and calculations" upon the performance of the marriage contract. But who has ever been able to calculate the course of a life? Mill's father, James Mill, may have called his first child into existence with the idea of making him a model soldier in the cause of Reform, but if so he miscalculated, for John Stuart Mill broke with the creed of his father—the essay *On Liberty* itself, both in manner and matter, recording his departure from those stark principles. After John Stuart, James Mill went on having one child

[*133*]

after another, not all of them, certainly, intended for ideological soldiers. It became the eldest child's resented duty to instruct the younger ones, and when John Stuart Mill records in his *Autobiography* that once he began learning Latin, "other sisters and brothers [were] successively added" as his own pupils, we detect beneath the flat statement a note of bewildered disgust with his father for doing something so completely contrary to reason, and contrary in particular to James Mill's heavy emphasis on temperance and belief that human life is barely worth having at all, as fathering one child after another. Adding more lives to an already unhappy world does not seem calculated to increase the sum of happiness. Writing to his son Pantagruel, Gargantua extols the power of reproduction as the most excellent gift bestowed on humanity by its divine creator. The younger Mill can say why people should not have children—"the consequence of their indulgence is a life or lives of wretchedness and depravity to the offspring"—but not why they ever should.

And this issue remains with us. Observed Christopher Lasch two decades ago,

> Psychiatrists who tell parents not to live through their children; married couples who postpone or reject parenthood, often for good practical reasons; social reformers who urge zero population growth, all testify to a pervasive uneasiness about reproduction—to widespread doubts, indeed, about whether our society should reproduce itself at all.

"Does making babies make sense?" asked a local ethicist, herself a mother. If an act makes sense only if calculated to promote the greatest happiness of the greatest number, the answer will be no. But if people are not born as a result of meticulous calculations of benefits, we can nevertheless imagine people putting an end to their lives as a result of calculation. An American today who believed doctrinally in the greatest happiness of the greatest number might consider his own life a robbery of resources from the world's poor. Some do talk this way, if only as an affectation. But imagine an elderly parent, a drain on the children's resources and a cause of much hardship and guilt, and conscious of all of this. In such a case the very act of calculation points toward suicide. You need only follow the numbers.

Besides this, if the ideal of "disengaged" reason calls for detachment from certain habits and desires with the purpose of "doing away" with them, isn't doing away with one's life the breaking of a habit par excellence? Suicide is the ultimate act of disengagement. Taunting Ivan Karamazov with his own vision of a heroic race of men who "accept death proudly and serenely like a god," the devil of his imagination is in fact the obscure double of Smerdyakov, who hanged himself moments before. A vision of Promethean self-conquest translates in practice into an act of covert revenge against the Karamazov family and a final statement of the hatred of life.

OF SOME we might say that keeping up with the fashions, political and otherwise, is for them a matter of life and death. Portraying as it does a man who meets his death as a consequence of decorating his house in the current fashion, *The Death of Ivan Ilych* offers a ruthlessly satiric example of such a person in action. The support groups that have swept the cancer world like some compelling psychological fashion are believed by some to be a matter of life and death, literally; hence the kind of study finding that "women with breast cancer who took part in support groups survived significantly longer than women who didn't attend." Defy the trend at the peril of your life. But perhaps the power of fashion really can extend to death.

I once heard a doctor voice his concern that physician-assisted suicide in the Netherlands was far too common and on the way to becoming a kind of moral fashion, as the duty of the old and the sick to relieve their families of their care catches on. Suicide in such cases presents itself as the last best expression of the ethos of self-mastery, humane concern, and rational calculation. But if the doctor is right, it can also be interpreted as the last word in political etiquette, the final act of one who dreads not doing the enlightened thing. In More's Utopia, one who is incurably ill is visited by priests and public officials who

> urge the invalid not to endure such agony any more. They remind him that he is now unfit for any of life's duties, a burden to himself and to others; he has really outlived his own death. . . . Those who have been persuaded by these arguments either starve themselves to death or take a potion which puts them painlessly to sleep.

No one has to argue Ivan Ilych into dying, nor is his decision to die authorized by any priest. But we can imagine a society where people *are* convinced to die—not by friendly persuaders bearing down on them in the name of religion and their own good, but simply by the voice of enlightened opinion. Already the "duty to die" is a term of social policy.

THE DEATH OF IVAN ILYCH:
THE LIMITS OF KNOWLEDGE

FOR ALL THE POWER of medicine itself and medical tools like the x-ray and the CT scan, much about the disease of cancer, including its causes and cure or cures, remains unknown. A good doctor approaches the disease in a spirit of uncertainty—not the paralyzing uncertainty of complete doubt but the sort that keeps you aware of the limits of knowledge. In the world of literature, the questions of what we know and how we know come to the fore in the novel, so much so that the novel itself might be called the narrative form of incomplete knowledge. The reader of a novel is presumed subject to error, uncertainty, and surprise, and the great novelists—high among them Tolstoy—manage these forces with great skill and power. Even *The Death of Ivan Ilych,* written in language that seems to know everything, leaves us with a respect for the unknown. It testifies to the incalculable in human affairs. While Tolstoy weaves into his tale a definite strain of Rousseau and relentlessly exposes sham and delusion, the net effect of all this isn't to render the world completely transparent but—almost to the contrary—to remind us of the poverty of our knowledge and to humble us before the unknowable. Writes Montaigne in his reflections on illness, Nature "keeps her processes absolutely unknown." So it is in *The Death of Ivan Ilych*. It is because they can't bear to admit that they have no idea what is going on inside him that Ivan Ilych's doctors torture him with their lies, their tests, their treatments. But not only the mechanism of disease—evidently some fast-moving cancer—lies concealed from human inquiry. So do the sources of revolt and the seeds of awakening.

The Death of Ivan Ilych opens with the report of the hero's death in the form of a pretentious obituary published by his wife, and interested comment by friends eyeing his now-vacant post. The atmosphere of sordid insincerity carries over to the memorial service in the hero's home, with the wife exploring the possibility of a fatter pension and the friends going through the motions of mourning, disturbed by the proximity of death and eager to resume their card games. The hypocrisy of these proceedings is laid bare by the author with the severity that distinguishes the entire work. We are so repelled by the sight of mourners profaning the solemnity of death with their parodies of grief that we cannot imagine the dead man himself was just as shallow and self-centered; all the more because "the expression on [his] face said that what was necessary had been accomplished, and accomplished rightly. Besides this there was in that expression a reproach and a warning to the living." As it happens, in life Ivan Ilych was morally indistinguishable from his false friends, and, had he been the survivor, he could easily have put in an appearance at a memorial for one of them on the way to an evening of cards, instead of the reverse. As Gary Saul Morson argues, Tolstoy is the master of "sideshadowing," the intimation of what might have happened if things had taken another turn. The fragility of the outcome of events in *The Death of Ivan Ilych* is itself a powerful fact whose significance dawns on the reader only slowly. In the reconstruction of the life of Ivan Ilych that follows the observance of his death, the turning point of the story—the onset of his reversal of fortune—is in fact the merest accident. He slips on a stepladder while hanging drapes. In its own anti-medical way, the tale of Ivan Ilych thus registers something like "the pervasive role of chance" in cancer.

In another work, such a misstep might be read as a symbol of the false path the hero has taken, or the perils of the ladder of success, but here the event is recounted so incidentally, with such a complete absence of portent or mystery, that only in retrospect does it stand out as the origin of the hero's illness. If a slip on a stepladder marks his tragic fall, this fall—maybe the most derisive in literature—also dramatizes his unfitness for the tragic role itself in the classical sense. Anyway, Ivan Ilych's careerism is plain enough without being italicized for the knowing reader by the special language of symbols. The son of a civil servant described in Dickensian terms as a "superfluous member of various superfluous institutions," Ivan Ilych follows the fashions of his class, attending law school, securing an official post, indulging in a little dissipation, and with the reform of the courts in the 1860s becoming an examining magistrate. In this position he learns the art of professionalism, screening out all but the official aspects of the case before him. He marries; almost at once, the marriage curdles. Just as he separates his personal views from official duties, he flees an odious domestic life by throwing himself into his work. Promoted to public prosecutor, he holds the position for some seven years, enjoying his power and more particularly the illusion of relief from the misery of his marriage. Three of his children have died.

Later, his career stagnating, Ivan Ilych journeys to St. Petersburg "with the sole object of obtaining a post with a salary of five thousand rubles a year." By good luck he finds such a place in his former department, where as an added delight he is now the superior of his old colleagues—a detail that brings out the atmosphere of petty comparisons in which he and his set live. It is at the zenith of his fortunes, while he is decorating a new house for his wife and daughter, that Ivan Ilych suffers the bruise in his side that marks the starting point of his ordeal. Over and beyond his physical pain is the moral torture, first of being treated by medical charlatans with the same haughty air he puts on in court (he too has become a case), second of being unable, practically until his last hour, to comprehend how it is that on his very deathbed he should be surrounded by pretenders.

At the end comes realization. Recognizing that his own life was the fraud he can now perceive so clearly in others, he is set free by the truth. As compassion even for his wife overcomes him, he dies to ease his family's sufferings as well as his own. Perhaps the look on the dead man's face said he had done his dying well because that is exactly what took place. A prisoner of false consciousness breaks through to the truth. A petty man performs an act of nobility.

In some plain sense of the word corresponding to the work's own repudiation of technical language, the story of Ivan Ilych is indeed a tragedy. He rises to a position of power and prosperity only to undergo the most complete humiliation and the most grueling suffering. The state of acceptance in which he dies, and which appears to be written on his face in death, constitutes tragic knowledge. But tragedy in this tale is subject to a double qualification. First, contrary to the tradition of drama itself, nothing happens suddenly in the tale, nothing disrupts the natural pace of time or vio-

lates the norms of common experience. Second, a mediocrity like Ivan Ilych, a mid-level civil servant, does not possess classical tragic stature. On his way to recognition, Ivan Ilych asks himself if it can really be possible that "I lost my life over that curtain as I might have done storming a fort." A tragic hero by any canonical definition does not hang curtains, still less give up his life doing so. That Ivan Ilych does lose his life as a result of an accident on a step-ladder—the contrary of a dramatic catastrophe, a nonevent of the same order as his widow's shawl catching on the edge of a table—vividly illustrates what Lionel Trilling calls the "absurdly *conditioned*" nature of daily life, so mortifying to human pride, as well as the folly of "the small concerns of this world." On the other hand, there is no getting away from daily life, and if Ivan Ilych deludes his own intelligence in decorating a house as though the life lived within its walls were not itself indecorous, he also deludes himself time and again by supposing he can shake off the prosaic facts of his domestic existence like dust off his feet. If we find our circumstances absurd and humiliating, this is precisely because they permit no escape. Only a Quixote dreams of attacking castles. Considered in the light of the prosaic, the idea of storming forts may in fact be just as hollow as that of beautifying an ugly life with the right drapes. (Considering that Ivan Ilych met disaster hanging drapes, it is especially ironic that his death should be degraded to the level of chitchat about sturgeon and "curtains.") An incongruous hero, Ivan Ilych is both more and less free than a classically tragic figure: more in as much as he is not subject to Fate or otherworldly agents (making his ruin absolutely his own doing), less in as much as he is subject to material necessities, embarrassments of the body, absurd conditions, traps of prosaic existence from which the other is exempt.

If the truth uncovered by Ivan Ilych in the course of his ordeal compares in horror to Oedipus's discovery that his entire life has been plotted, this is in part because his own life was scripted as well. Where Tolstoy's art shatters the model of tragic composition, Ivan Ilych follows the way of life laid down by his class as implicitly as if he were obeying an edict of destiny, even marrying because it seems the correct thing to do. Like Oedipus, that is, he walks blindly into the lethal trap that has been prepared for him, except that it has been prepared not by Fate but by the human beings whose ways he imitates, the members of good society. That the story line he follows to his own ruin was written not by the gods but by mortals as deluded as himself makes his subjection to it all the more absurd and pitiful. Walking straight into a cage "from which there was no way of escape," Ivan Ilych provides an illustration all at once prosaic, tragic, and ridiculous of the dictum that man, born free, is everywhere in chains.

FOR THE MOST PART, the implications of his own actions descend on Ivan Ilych as suffering follows crime in the logic of tragedy—except that in this case all is the work of natural causality, not avenging furies or the decrees of law. Try as he may to escape his wife, Ivan Ilych must return to her vulgarity sooner or later and reckon with the humiliations he brought on himself when he married her. Try as he may to ignore, arrest, or even palliate his disease (the result of another misstep, in this case literal), it returns with full force. That he experiences at the hands of his physicians exactly the sort of almightiness he himself radiates in court may seem the work of a retributive God but is actually the natural consequence of his own fascination with illusory goods like celebrity and prestige. In-

stead of haunting specters and inescapable edicts, Ivan Ilych is subjected to the haunting returns of his own actions and the bitter futility of the attempt to escape from himself.

So it is that the horror of his story as he himself comes to understand it lies not so much in how he dies as in how he lived. Even his decorating accident would not have happened had he not been so intent on outfitting his house with "all the things people of a certain class have in order to resemble other people of that class." The accident itself is the kind of thing that could well happen within the ordinary course of events—something, as it were, minimally improbable. Like the machinery of the supernatural, the wonders of romance are rigorously excluded as violations of the work's intent to bring the hero to an examination of his own life without distractions or excuses. The expedient used to achieve this end is the most natural one possible, the furthest from the artifices of fiction: illness. Immobilizing him, isolating him from practically all other human souls but the loyal servant Gerasim (of whom more later), illness leaves Ivan Ilych with no release from suffering and nothing to do but think. That his doctors prove to be his mirror image is anything but a coincidence. The allure of social brilliance that drew him to his wife in the first place, and draws her to Sarah Bernhardt as he lies dying, also makes her insist on his consulting "a celebrated doctor" at the onset of his illness, and it is this notable who treats him with the same show of superiority he himself puts on in court. From Ivan Ilych's experience of this impostor come the first rays of enlightenment—not only a sense of what the wretches in his own power might feel but a dim perception of his own falsity, now glimpsed in another. Precisely in their arrogance and fraud, the doctors in *The Death of Ivan Ilych* serve as the catalysts of the hero's awakening. Ivan Ilych is linked to these tormentors as closely as a

man and his own reflection, almost as closely as the terms of a syllogism. Only in seeking again and again to evade his condition does Ivan Ilych learn it cannot be evaded, and only by entangling himself in delusion is he brought face to face with his capacity for self-deceit.

Guilty of killing his father and marrying his mother but without the knowledge that these are his parents, Oedipus defines the tragic conundrum of guilt-in-innocence that applies as well to Ivan Ilych. The case of Ivan Ilych is of a different kind, however, in that he commits no crime, no real act of turpitude, nothing that seems to justify the ordeal of his slow death. "But I'm not guilty!" he cries out some weeks before the end, his struggle not yet concluded, and in a narrow sense he is correct. As a judge he never took bribes or threw people in jail for no reason, "never abused his power; on the contrary he tried to soften its expression." Scrupulous and incorruptible even as he tempers justice with mercy, Ivan Ilych seems more like a textbook example of a good judge than one who deserves to be tried and convicted himself. He lives by the book of propriety as well, marrying because it is what decent people do and following the social code in all things. In point of fact it is the outward irreproachability of Ivan Ilych's life that constitutes his guilt in the author's eyes and at last in his own. Though passing at his ease through crowds of supplicants in the enjoyment of his power (again somewhat in the manner of Oedipus) violates no statute, the act is indecent. Under the sanction of legal propriety Ivan Ilych treats those in his power with a kind of majesty whose fraudulence he can appreciate only when he experiences the same thing at the hands of his detested doctors; under the cover of social convention he leads a domestic life so sordid it verges on the obscene. In either case it is the knowledge that he is abiding by an established code of conduct

that allows him to act so unreflectively. Innocence underwrites indecency and fraud. As if in a free interpretation of the intermediate character of the tragic hero, Ivan Ilych is neither admirable nor depraved, and suitably to the satiric logic of tragedy, the very principles in which he found his safety prove his ruin.

And so he endures not only great suffering but a kind of absolute abasement. Subjected to tragedy's mocking logic, he finds his own power of action turned against him and must try himself where before he tried others. The reversal of his fortunes brings with it recognition—in this instance, recognition of his own falsity. Also as in the case of a tragic hero, Ivan Ilych is by no means the worst of men in spite of his sins, and his torment seems in excess of justice. But this is tragedy with a cardinal difference, Tolstoy having eliminated the most axiomatic quality of the tragic hero, the source of all his other qualities, his singularity. In the world of Oedipus there is none like him. Another of his magnitude would be a second sun in the heavens. Tragic greatness tolerates no rivals. Like a figure raised above the ground, it stands out against everything else, now reduced by contrast to a single plane. The same sort of naturalism that leads Tolstoy to do nothing by jumps in *The Death of Ivan Ilych,* but instead to trace the gradual working of great changes, prohibits a hero who has vaulted beyond the ordinary range of human character and experience. At least until the onset of his crisis, nothing sets Ivan Ilych morally apart from the friends who hasten from his memorial to their card game (he himself loved cards), the doctors who impose to the very end, possibly even the wife who leaves him on his sickbed to take in the performance of Sarah Bernhardt. The hero of this tragedy—the creation of a resolutely prosaic imagination—is made of the same stuff as the most base.

According to Aristotle, tragedy excites pity and fear—pity for unmerited suffering and fear for "the person like us." In Ivan Ilych this latter condition becomes absolute. Tolstoy has fashioned one so completely like us as to shatter the Aristotelian paradigm, a man indistinguishable from any other of his sort until he literally stumbles onto tragic experience. Ironized in Ivan Ilych is the very salience of a hero, that quality in virtue of which all eyes fasten onto him. Hanging drapes in an attempt to give his new house a touch of salience, he succeeds only in making it look "so like others that it would never have been noticed, but to him it all seemed to be quite exceptional." Thinking himself a figure, Ivan Ilych proves himself a nobody. In one sense, however, this lack of singularity may be a virtue. Those in *The Death of Ivan Ilych* who play up their own distinction, whether eminent doctors or the great Sarah Bernhardt or the also theatrical Praskovya Fedorovna in her role as the queen of suffering—all appear as corrupt and fraudulent as the theater itself in the opinion of Rousseau. Such is the originality of *The Death of Ivan Ilych* that it constitutes a tragedy, and a great one, even as it rejects theatricality per se and exposes the dramatization of the self as the cultivation of a false distinction.

As it turns out, the warning written on Ivan Ilych's face in death is therefore directed at those no different from himself. First meeting him as he lies in state, we cannot imagine that the life he led was completely out of character with his postmortem dignity. The sage in death was a fool in life. That he did break through his own delusions means, however, that the power of sham over him was not absolute. Is it not possible, then, that some other trifler or opportunist will one day break through as well, even if it be in the shadow of death? So stereotypical are Ivan Ilych's false friends and insincere wife that we cannot begin to envision them awakening to their own disgrace as he does. But he did awaken, and who is to say they cannot? It is true that they seem the very definition of hypocrisy, as though hypocrisy summed up their entire being and they could never become other than who they are. But a careerist is all Ivan Ilych gave any appearance of being. For Schwartz with his false cheer or Praskovya Fedorovna with her addiction to acting and aversion to truth to look into themselves is not so much more unlikely than the thought of Ivan Ilych, a man of no originality, disowning the script he lived by. If it was as a result of his childhood that some flicker of truth remained with Ivan Ilych in adult life, had not others a childhood? In spite of his escapism, there is already a momentary glint of awareness, a stirring of possibility, in the hero's friend Peter Ivanovich, distressed as he is at the "consciousness of his own and [Praskovya Fedorovna's] dissimulation" at the dead man's memorial. The detail appears incidentally and passes quickly, as the report of Ivan Ilych's misstep does also.

Dostoevsky was not alone in appreciating that "man is not a final and defined quantity upon which firm calculations can be made, man is free, and can therefore violate any regulating norms which might be thrust upon him," for who would calculate that one so hollow as Ivan Ilych, so incapable as it seems of reflection, would find it in himself to put his own existence into question? But if the seeming nonentity Ivan Ilych possesses the tragic spark, so might others equally unpromising. In this tragedy in opposition to Aristotle, precisely because the hero is ordinary (as is the incident that triggers his crisis) someone else could conceivably occupy his position. What of the fop engaged to his daughter, like himself an examining magistrate? What of the coachman he had as a child or the "various shabby friends and relations" who at one time descended on his household? In this world the center of consciousness can be anywhere. Though he does not probe the limits of Euclidean reality like his mighty opposite Dostoevsky, Tolstoy does open up the Aristotelian framework by depriving the tragic hero of his primary possession, his uniqueness.

At the time of his accident, no sign appears of what is truly remarkable in Ivan Ilych, his power to question and reflect. But if this man seemingly without distinction carries within himself the seed of tragic capacity and the potential for enlightenment, may not others as well? What if the tale contains stirrings of meaning we do not yet register, just as Ivan Ilych's stumble reads as his "downfall" only after the fact? Before the significance of that event was perfectly obvious, it was perfectly invisible. On his deathbed it occurs to Ivan Ilych that "his scarcely perceptible attempts to struggle against what was considered good by the most highly placed people, those scarcely noticeable impulses which he had immediately suppressed, might have been the real thing, and all the rest false." Maybe other signs in the tale go unrecognized as well. After all, Gerasim, who leaps into prominence in the latter part of the work, barely attracts our notice in its first section. Another background figure, Ivan Ilych's son Vasya, is a kind of crux of indeterminacy, possessing as he does something of the beauty of childhood even though, at his father's memorial, his eyes have the look of "boys of thirteen or fourteen who are not pure-minded." What will this schoolboy become? We might think of *The Death of Ivan Ilych* as a detective story with no crime in the conventional sense, with clues of the highest subtlety, but most important—and in accordance with Tolstoy's own distrust of the neatness of narrative—with an open solution.

ONE EVENING while Ivan Ilych lies dying, his wife enters the room dressed to the nines, "her full bosom pushed up by her corset, and with traces of powder on her face. She had reminded him in the morning that they were going to the theater. Sarah Bernhardt was visiting town." In her shallowness and grotesque sensuality, Praskovya Fedorovna serves as a living illustration of Rousseau's thesis of the depraving effect of the theater and of good society itself. Just as Ivan Ilych's loss of happiness and entrapment in falsity pick up Rousseau's theme of the fatal effect of dependence on public opinion (and it is Rousseau, after all, whose maxim "Man is born free; and is everywhere in chains" presides like a sort of warning inscription over *The Death of Ivan Ilych*), so it was the purely social brilliance deplored by Rousseau that attracted Ivan Ilych to this woman in the first place. Tolstoy, we are reminded,

> remained an admirer of Rousseau, and late in life still recommended *Émile* as the best book ever written on education. Rousseau must have strengthened, if he did not actually originate, his growing tendency to idealise the soil and its cultivators—the simple peasant, who for Tolstoy is a repository of almost as rich a stock of "natural" virtues as Rousseau's noble savage.

The simple peasant is exemplified in *The Death of Ivan Ilych* in the butler's assistant, whose kindly offices to the dying man contrast so sharply with the selfishness of his wife. For her part, in attempting to parlay her husband's death into a fatter pension, Praskovya Fedorovna, like the friends interested in the dead man's post, displays a glaring lack of Rousseauvian virtue, for it was a principle with Rousseau "never to profit in any way by the death of anyone dear to me." Praskovya Fedorovna stands before us fully defined, the very type of vanity and luxury in the complete Rousseauvian sense. That is what she is, and that is all she will ever be. Confirming to the letter Rousseau's portrayal of the falsity of those goods that exist only in the eyes of society, she possessed charm as a girl and is drawn to prestige in the person of renowned doctors and celebrity in that of Sarah Bernhardt. In complaining, during the memorial for her husband, of how greatly she suffered at the end, her theatrics are of one piece with the falsity she displayed in quitting him for the theater in the first place. This woman is a known quantity. She is the human image of insincerity and will never be anything other than that. It is impossible to read *The Death of Ivan Ilych* without a strong conviction that this is the interpretation the author intends.

But the tale itself plays the fox to the author's intention.

For much as Ivan Ilych outgrows what seems like his own fixed nature, achieving tragic stature and insight, so the tale itself transcends the ideological framework so forcibly stamped upon it by the author's Rousseauvian program. If Praskovya Fedorovna stands fully defined, her husband once seemed locked into his definition as a nonentity—a man of no depth, a hopeless prisoner of false consciousness—and that impression itself proved false. Whatever the intent of the teller, the tale itself shows that our experience cannot be predetermined, our moral capacities known with finality in advance of experience. In short, no one is really an open book. Of none can it be said with certainty: this person is forever incapable of enlightenment. That Ivan Ilych dies asking his wife's forgiveness, overcome with pity at the sight of her suffering, establishes Praskovya Fedorovna in any case as more than a caricature of a human being. Throughout the tale she has figured as a kind of degrading circumstance Ivan Ilych cannot escape—the shackle on his foot. In the end the richly prosaic imagination of Tolstoy cannot reduce this daughter of commonplace beneath the level of humanity. Through the last act of Ivan Ilych, the definition of Praskovya Fedorovna as a common shrew, and nothing but that, is retracted.

It is said that Tolstoy in *War and Peace* "wanted to change our habit of viewing our lives as if they resembled conventional narratives. Our lives have not been authored in advance, but are lived as we go along. They are process, not product." The iconoclastic spirit of this project—the revolt against conventional narrative as if it were one more means of bewitching human intelligence, like the mysteries of freemasonry or priestcraft—is probably responsible for the independence of *The Death of Ivan Ilych* itself, that is, the complete freedom with which it handles the principles of tragedy. But if lives are not authored in advance, neither is the outcome of the life story of Ivan Ilych's false friends, or even his detestable wife, given in advance. Tolstoy indeed categorizes relentlessly, so relentlessly that even characters at the fringes of the tale, like the various unnamed "shabby friends and relations" who descend on Ivan Ilych at one point "with much show of affection," seem to wear their definition on their brow. Tolstoy's word renders summary judgment. But as the tale of Ivan Ilych unfolds, Tolstoy's deed contradicts his word. Here is a man displayed before us like a specimen in a case, categorized as a blind fool, who transcends his own typicality in the ordeal of coming to consciousness. The extraordinary fact of his awakening calls into question the dismissive characterization of all the others in the tale categorized scarcely more summarily than himself. Their history remains unwritten. Under the tale's non-Aristotelian conditions, no one figure engrosses all tragic potential. Others too may achieve the dignity of tragic stature—who, how, and when we cannot say. "Contingency always reigns," as it reigned

over Ivan Ilych's mishap in the first place. If Ivan Ilych—Anyman—
is thrust into the heroic position by chance and achieves, over time,
insight he could never have been imagined capable of, one equally
improbable may also at some time be ennobled by suffering. (The
drawing-out of time in *The Death of Ivan Ilych* brings to mind the
description of the long latency period for cancer as "giving time for
the improbable to happen.") By analogy with the richness of character that makes it impossible to reduce Ivan Ilych to an overpaid
bureaucrat, the tale as such possesses a profound humanity that takes
it out of conformity with the narrow views behind it.

WHO, other than Ivan Ilych, might be capable of moral awakening
cannot be known. *The Death of Ivan Ilych* is a testament to the unknowable. The doctors pretending to treat Ivan Ilych are marked as
frauds by their shows of knowledge. So great, in fact, is Tolstoy's suspicion of false knowledge that he is willing to dismiss medicine as
an institution. When Natasha falls ill, of moral causes, in *War and
Peace,*

> Doctors came to see her singly and in consultation, talked
> much in French, German, and Latin, blamed one another, and
> prescribed a great variety of medicines for all the diseases
> known to them, but the simple idea never occurred to any of
> them that they could not know the disease Natasha was suf-
> fering from, as no disease suffered by a live man can be
> known, for every living person has his own peculiarities and
> always has his own peculiar, personal, novel, complicated dis-
> ease, unknown to medicine—not a disease of the lungs, liver,
> skin, heart, nerves, and so on mentioned in medical books, but

a disease consisting of one of the innumerable combinations of the maladies of those organs. This simple thought could not occur to the doctors (as it cannot occur to a wizard that he is unable to work charms) because the business of their lives was to cure, and they received money for it and had spent the best years of their lives on that business.

Even while the doctors try to determine if the trouble lies in his kidney or his appendix, Ivan Ilych is dying of some disease that eludes medicine altogether. Apparently, though, it was the bruise to his side that activated his disease or brought all of its elements into play, and to this extent *The Death of Ivan Ilych* supports the social theory of disease. Ivan Ilych dies because he wanted his drapes hung just so—dies of his way of life. (The peasant Gerasim, living a healthy life, is shown in health.) From the triggering event and the judgment it renders on his life to the fraudulent treatment he receives in the name of medicine, the portrayal of Ivan Ilych's illness is filled with satiric scorn, disgust, ridicule, and cruelty. How is it, then, that in spite of Tolstoy's wrath and his indictment of medicine as an organized fraud, *The Death of Ivan Ilych* speaks profoundly even to our own age of medical advances? The answer must be that just as the tale rises above its own narrow ideological program—its condemnation of good society, its caricature of woman, its dismissal of law—so too does its depiction of suffering transcend the author's harsh prejudice against medicine itself. And this is a measure of its greatness.

OVER RECENT MONTHS, *The Death of Ivan Ilych* has never been far from my mind. According to the view of certain cancer coun-

selors, however, this great tale would simply stand for the dark traditions that enslave us and even keep us sick. Write two such counselors:

> There is no courtroom judge that is stricter than the one that
> may be inside you. The cultural myth supports this self-
> judgment since cancer is often seen as a judgment or punish-
> ment for wrongdoing. It is like the story of Job in the Bible in
> which all of Job's friends tell him he must have done some-
> thing wrong to cause his misfortunes. The sense of guilt that
> can accompany cancer can keep you small and prevent you
> from imagining yourself free of cancer.

It is almost as though these words were directed at Tolstoy's tale of
a judge who judges himself, in the process recognizing how he
brought on his own fatal illness. In the eyes of the counselors, this
work of incomparable power and bitter irony could only be a fal-
lacy, an expression of a particularly vicious myth, an example of the
Old Law abolished by the new way of therapy. The replacement of
depth and power by vapidity follows unavoidably from the reduction of our tradition to a legacy of ignorance and myth.

SMALL OFFICES OF KINDNESS

![ornament] IN CONTRAST to a more classical figure, the character at the center of Tolstoy's tragedy seems to be a man of no distinction at all, an accidental hero. As boldly as Peter Brueghel's *Landscape with the Fall of Icarus,* this tale ironizes the very principle of centrality. Where Brueghel relegates to an insignificant corner of the painting the sensational event of a boy's fall from the sky, only to concentrate on a plowman doing nothing out of the ordinary, the prosaic Tolstoy has his hero die not as the result of a sensational event like storming a fort, but a loss of footing—an event so perfectly ordinary it scarcely registers *as* an event. In the same way, and in keeping with his revaluation of importance itself, Tolstoy brings forward in the course of the tale a figure at first camouflaged as a background character of no particular significance: the butler's assistant Gerasim. "Only rarely," writes Iris Murdoch at the very end of *The Sovereignty of Good,* "does one meet somebody in whom [humility] positively shines, in whom one apprehends with amazement the absence of the anxious avaricious tentacles of the self." Such a person is Gerasim.

Gerasim is the faithful plowman of *The Death of Ivan Ilych,* doing his work well even in the presence of death. When we meet

Gerasim at the memorial service for Ivan Ilych (whose wife, like some incarnation of avarice, is thinking of her pension), he is first seen "strewing something on the floor" and later helping Peter Ivanovich with his coat. In reply to Peter Ivanovich's inept remark, "Well, friend Gerasim. It's a sad affair, isn't it?" Gerasim answers,

> "It's God's will. We shall all come to it some day," [and displays] his teeth—the even, white teeth of a healthy peasant—and like a man in the thick of urgent work, he briskly opened the front door, called the coachman, helped Peter Ivanovich into the sledge, and sprang back to the porch as if in readiness for what he had to do next.

At this point in the tale no reader could possibly envision the role this servant will play as the comforter of Ivan Ilych. If he calls no attention to himself (unlike the hero's wife, who loves theatrics and dramatizes her own false suffering), neither does Tolstoy draw any particular attention to Gerasim.

The doctors are unable to comfort Ivan Ilych except by drugging him, just as priestcraft or freemasonry drugs human intelligence, according to the author's ideas. Gerasim is able to comfort Ivan Ilych simply by doing what is asked of him: raising his master's legs.

> [Ivan Ilych] saw that no one felt for him, because no one even wished to grasp his position. Only Gerasim recognized it and pitied him. And so Ivan Ilych felt at ease only with him. He felt comforted when Gerasim supported his legs (sometimes all night long) and refused to go to bed, saying, "Don't you worry, Ivan Ilych. I'll get sleep enough later on," or, when he suddenly became familiar and exclaimed: "If you weren't sick it would

be another matter, but as it is, why should I grudge a little trouble?" Only Gerasim did not lie; everything showed that he alone understood the facts of the case and did not consider it necessary to disguise them, but simply felt sorry for his emaciated and enfeebled master.

"The humble man," says Iris Murdoch, "because he sees himself as nothing, can see other things as they are." Gerasim's candor, of course, stands in the sharpest contrast to the mendacity of Ivan Ilych's doctors.

In the course of treatment I encountered no impostors but many Gerasims—nurses and technicians who worked in the background and never seemed to expect recognition, certainly never sent a bill, performers of the small offices of kindness that have no insurance codes but come between the patient and misery. The indignities of prostate cancer are like those of age itself (how different from the Shakespearean canker that destroys "the infants of the spring"), with the refinement in my own case that age came before its time. Somewhat like Ivan Ilych with his mishap on a stepladder, or his wife with her caught shawl, I got caught in some painful absurdities. About these some of my Gerasims joked and some didn't, but none pretended that nothing of the kind was happening. When I was reduced to humiliation—filling with urine I couldn't seem to void—the response of my Gerasims was always to acknowledge the fact with good humor, like their Tolstoyan counterpart, and do what they could. Like Gerasim himself, alert for what he had to do next, the Gerasims of my experience were doers. They used duct tape as well as rubber bands, and for the sake of those who looked up from a metal table, flat on their backs, put stars on the ceiling.

The joker of the group was undoubtedly the rubber-band

artist. When, after a lengthy ordeal, he finally got all the ultrasound images the medical physicist would need for his computations, he printed out one more. "Here," said the wag, handing over an image of my own prostate. "Send it as a Christmas card." In context this meant: "The images came out well, and thank God it's over."

For all his hatred of medicine, Tolstoy himself might have appreciated this Gerasim. It was because the standard way of doing the job simply didn't work that he had to resort to rubber bands. In fact, he implied, the standard way never works. "You can throw out the textbook," he said. In that remark Tolstoy's entire philosophy of history and narrative is encapsulated.

IN AN ESSAY already cited here, the author, a breast-cancer patient, seems to feel nothing but resentment and scorn toward the few nurses and technicians mentioned, as if she were too angry to experience gratitude. Not that resentment and gratitude are just alternative expressions of ardor, one precluding the other. People do not, I believe, have a grateful mentality in the way many do have a resentful mentality, possessed of a general sense of injury, predisposed to ill-will and accusation, their minds bathed in the acid of antipathy. We speak of a resentful person but not so naturally of a grateful person. In addition, resentment can be directed toward abstract objects more readily than gratitude. Gratitude remembers a favor, a joke, a mode of address, warm blankets, stuck-on stars, a bottle of juice. A patient who blames her plight on "the corporations" seems too possessed with abstract objects to be mindful of the small services of a nurse or technician—figures portrayed in this case as agents of an alien system. By the same token, I cannot imagine hating an abstract object with the particularity of gratitude.

CRUEL CHOICES

TOLSTOY LIKENED *War and Peace* to the *Iliad.* The hero of the *Iliad* itself, Achilles, has a choice between two destinies: achieving fame by dying at Troy or enjoying a long life.

> If I stay here and fight beside the city of the Trojans,
> my return home is gone but my glory shall be everlasting;
> but if I return home to the beloved land of my fathers,
> the excellence of my glory is gone, but there will be a long
>   life
> left for me.

Perhaps it's an index of the more romantic and wishful nature of the *Odyssey* that its hero achieves fame without dying for it and is even promised by the prophet Tiresias "a sleek old age." Odysseus is the original survivor. He too faces hard choices, though, as between Scylla and Charybdis. (It is revealing that we sometimes speak of "sailing between Scylla and Charybdis," the one option Odysseus does not have.) No doubt whenever we choose between two things we forgo one for the other, but in certain cases we are forced to decide, and the stakes of decision are high. With Achilles the choice is between nothing less than two paths that might be symbolized by the unnamed plowman who lives out his unremarkable life and the boy Icarus who earned fame through death—a distinction corresponding to that between fidelity to the prosaic and, on the other hand, the idealization of "extreme moments" and the belief in "the revelatory power of the extraordinary."

A choice as stark, as unavoidable, and as fateful as Achilles' is put to the reader of Machiavelli. As Isaiah Berlin explains,

> One is obliged to choose: and in choosing one form of life, give up the other. That is the central point. If Machiavelli is right, . . . it is in principle impossible to be morally good and do one's duty as this was conceived by common European, and, especially, Christian ethics, and at the same time build Sparta or Periclean Athens or the Rome of the Republic or even of the Antonines.

We must decide between two contradictory goods, Christian virtue and the active life, both of which really are goods. If one were not, the choice would not be so hard or so significant. Whatever his reputation, Machiavelli does not love cruelty for its own sake, but the choice he leaves us with is cruel in itself. It is the master theme of Isaiah Berlin's thought that, as in this case, there is no way to reconcile all human goods.

Hard choices are things we prefer to evade. According to the Grand Inquisitor, if there is one thing human beings want more than another, it is to get rid of the power and burden of choice. The creator of the Grand Inquisitor, Ivan Karamazov, chooses neither to defend his father nor to kill him but simply to walk away at the moment of crisis, thinking he has thereby evaded the issue entirely but finding himself more entangled than ever.

Another way to slip the knot of hard choices is to pretend that a choice doesn't really have costs. Such are the costs of Achilles' choice of a glorious death that when Odysseus meets him in the underworld in the *Odyssey* he, Achilles, declares that he

> would rather follow the plow as thrall of another man, one
> with no land allotted him and not much to live on,
> than be a king over all the perished dead.

Even Achilles, it seems, would like to have it both ways. So do we all. Near the end of *A Doll's House,* Ibsen's famous heroine proclaims that her duty to her family is matched by an equally sacred duty to herself. She seems caught between competing principles of equal rank. Moments later, however, Nora asserts that her supreme obligation is to herself, and this being so, she can fulfill it without offending any principle equally important. Her bind unbinds itself. Accordingly, Nora is not seen tearing herself away from children and home but walking out, as though her revolt did not cost much.

It would be strange if the ideal of progress that has had such animating power over the past two centuries did not hold out the hope of lessening unbearable choices—of relieving the economics of scarcity dictating that we can have one necessary thing only at the expense of another. To John Stuart Mill, the contradiction posed by Machiavelli between Christian virtue and the active life does not exist. The two are complementary, together adding up to something greater than either. "Truth, in the great practical concerns of life," he writes in *On Liberty,* "is so much a question of the reconciling and combining of opposites. . . ." (Some refer to techniques like hydrotherapy as complementary medicine, as though they were the missing half of the medical art.) Albert O. Hirschman, in his study of the arguments used to thwart progress, attributes to the enemies of progress that belief that no good thing can be had but at the cost of another—the belief, for example, that the computer will extinguish the book, that the "rise" of one thing spells the "fall" of another. It is true that such claims are made and received without much thought. But so are claims that good things can't really conflict, precisely because they are good. Teach at an open-enrollment university and you will find that its admissions policy clashes with academic standards no matter how defined, but you will also find that this conflict—this massively obvious and inescapable conflict—officially does not exist. We like having the best of both worlds, SUVs both rugged and luxurious. Using anti-cancer ingredients, Michael Milken's chef simulates the taste of American favorites. "Chili. Reuben sandwiches. Strawberry short cake. It hardly seemed possible. I could eat well while undergoing nutrition therapy. I *could* have it both ways."

But that hard choices confront us doesn't mean that they call for some blind leap of the will. A choice well made is not made arbitrarily and definitely is not made in a spirit of fantasy, resentment, or despair, whatever the pull of these motives in ourselves or their accreditation in our culture. And as Iris Murdoch points out, we choose well "'when the time comes' not out of strength of will but out of the quality of our usual attachments," which is to say that behind dramatic choices stand background conditions, daily practices, habits of loyalty—the plowman at his work.

IN THE ABSENCE of a cure for prostate cancer, support groups have been advertised as a kind of talking cure for the disease's woes. It is said that when you join a support group, you learn that "you—like the other men in the group—have the power to manage your cancer and still lead a full and satisfying life." Properly coached, the man with cancer is like someone enjoying a good simulation of a Reuben sandwich: he can hardly tell the difference.

Misery loves company of course, but why is it that claims for the therapeutic benefits of support groups ring so false? "Attend a meeting and you will see that you don't have to go through this alone." Inches after this statement, the authors of *Prostate Cancer: What Every Man—and His Family—Needs to Know* caution that "the time will arrive when you, and you alone, must decide what to do." But what makes decisions about treatment painful isn't that they have to be made alone (in my case they were not), but that they are difficult in themselves—something like the choice of Achilles, except that for the prostate cancer patient there is certainly no glory and there may or may not be long life.

For the prostate cancer patient, doing one thing may preclude doing another, and this when no one quite knows what to do in the first place. Every choice is potentially costly. Elect "watchful waiting" and you may lose the possibility of treating the cancer when it is most treatable. Treat it and you may start down a slippery slope; in any case, you bring on yourself the likelihood of some ugly side effects and still have no certainty of cure. Nor do you necessarily make a hard choice once and get it over with. Seeds mitigate these dilemmas but do not dissolve them; nor are seeds an option in every case. (To reduce costs, seed implants are sometimes done in Veterans' Hospitals without imaging the prostate beforehand—in effect, done blind. For those who undergo this cut-rate treatment, the likelihood of eradicating the cancer must be lower and the side effects worse.) Some patients are eventually reduced to choosing impotence, though the counselors of good cheer assure them that "No matter what treatment you choose for prostate cancer, you can still be powerful, passionate, and sexy." Statements like that cover up harsh choices as though they were some kind of ideological embarrassment, a relic of the ages when people possessed of an archaic mentality supposed that choices had costs.

If others are like me, they may even be unaware of the choice before them, in part because of the very nature of publicity. In the case of prostate cancer, publicity inherently favors the active approach. Screenings after all have a lot more publicity value than the arguments against screening, arguments that sound like perverse inventions if you do get wind of them, so contrary are they to the usual public messages. The message that science cannot reliably distinguish lethal from dormant cancers doesn't lend itself to publicity campaigns and doesn't rouse people to action. Just as a mammogram bus claims more attention than questions over the value of mammography, so "Prostate Cancer Awareness" upstages the opposition, to the point that this patient never realized an opposition existed. The skeptics have nothing to match bright ribbons, community runs, and above all the rhetoric of saving lives.

In the case of breast cancer, the rhetoric of emergency creates the false impression that "all breast tumors will eventually kill us if left untreated and that catching them early is our only hope," in effect distracting us from our own ignorance. In the prostate cancer world you hear the same cries of "Fire!" In my own case, it was only after treatment that one of the doctors said I would have died within a few years had the disease taken its course. Certainly I do not regret treatment. What I regret is the presumption that the public as a whole, myself included, cannot make a difficult choice between alternatives and thus has to be spared the pain of deciding and presented with an absolute. Iris Murdoch argues that the school of philosophy reducing moral language to emotive utterances misrepresents the very nature of moral life. According to one such philosopher,

> Persuasion is not directed to a person as a rational agent, who is asking himself (or us) "What shall I do?"; it is not an answer to this or any other question; it is an attempt to *make* him answer it in a particular way.

As though we got the sort of language the prevailing philosophy bargains for, the public language of cancer often works exactly like this. It gets us to reply to a given question with a given answer.

At a higher level, a choice needs to be made between two visions of human life: one that affirms the very capacity for risk and responsibility as indispensable to human dignity; and a therapeutic worldview that pictures others as needing to be shielded from risk and responsibility, incapable somehow, "patients" and not agents—a worldview with a sort of vested interest in diminished capacity, more concerned that human beings do the healthy or the beneficial thing (as these words are predefined) than respectful of human independence. When a cancer researcher writes that in coming years

> it is likely that the cancer burden will become more focused . . . on the less privileged—in other words, on those less able or less well-equipped to take charge of their lives and make the informed choices available to the rest of us,

with the implication that someone qualified is obviously going to have to make their decisions for them, he does not even bother to consider the moral costs of declaring broad bands of the population incompetent—as though the therapeutic imperative were so urgent that no other principle could possibly rival it.

"IN POLITICS," writes John Stuart Mill, "it is almost a common-place, that a party of order or stability, and a party of progress or re-form, are both necessary elements of a healthy state of political life," the two being held in balance in a flourishing commonwealth. But in some domains it may not be possible to reconcile these compet-ing principles. The zeal for experiment, the rejection of limits, and indeed the drive to extend life that belong not only to a Michael Milken but to any modern moved by the spirit of progress and the emancipation of desire—how is this to be squared with traditional precepts of acceptance and submission, warnings against vain ambi-tion and excessive desire, the duty to bear well what must be borne, the principle of remaining within the limits binding upon us? In my view these mentalities conflict too completely to be balanced like rival interests in a robust state. We must choose between them. That might seem easy, especially as, being moderns, we take so readily to maxims of progress and so unreadily to those of stability. We are steeped in the theory of unlimited possibility. But of course we are also subject to limits, first and last the limits on life itself.

PUBLICITY AND
ENLIGHTENMENT

Vice could grow impudent, without becoming red with shame. Virtue knew no means of sharing its suffering, or gaining the sympathy of society. The law had no critics, morals had no supervisor, reason was monopolized. Providence spoke: let the human race become free! And "publicity" appeared.

—Wilhelm Wekhrlin (1784)

IT WAS Tolstoy's belief that no two cases of disease are alike, that "each unhealthy organism is unhealthy in its own way." In the case of cancer, there is some medical truth to this, it seems. "In a sense, every patient's cancer is unique. . . . In so far as it is a disease, [cancer] is a collection of very many (a thousand or so) disorders of cell and tissue function." Nevertheless, Tolstoy's view of disease as a deep and confounding mystery was not a medical intuition but, if you will, a satiric one. It is as if the great novelist overextended the satiric principle that experience alone can clear delusion, experience being something no one can acquire for another. Just as Ivan Ilych cannot transmit to another the lessons of his suffering, so experience belongs by definition to the one who has it, and illness represents a kind of heightening of experience. The singular Montaigne reflects on illness and medicine in his essay "On Experience." As experience belongs to a single person, so too is the ultimate focus of medical treatment a single person.

States the Hippocratic oath in part, "You do solemnly swear . . . that you will exercise your art solely for the cure of your patients." But of course this doesn't mean that physicians are to act for the benefit of their patients in general, still less of society in general. They are to act for the benefit of each patient, and surely most take that duty to heart. In an age when the responsibility *of* the individual has been thrown into question and in good part subverted by theories of causation and reluctance to judge, physicians have helped preserve responsibility *to* the individual. Some think the medical focus on the patient too narrow, too individualistic. For my part, I was relieved to be in the care of physicians who served no larger cause than my own, and as a gainer from their skill I looked with less favor on reformers who liken themselves to physicians— physicians to society itself.

Certain social scientists, casting their eyes on the achievements of natural science, are said to suffer from physics envy. The success of medicine has called forth physician envy; or at least the prestige of medicine has made that skill an irresistibly attractive source of metaphors and other rhetorical ornaments.

By the time Bentham portrayed himself as a physician ministering to the body politic, such imagery was already a convention of the Enlightenment. Locke was himself a physician, and "medicine had been intimately linked to the scientific revolution—which was at bottom a philosophical revolution—from the beginning; the pioneers of that revolution saw themselves as physicians to a sick civilization." To the thinkers of the Enlightenment, writes Peter Gay, revealed religion was a "sick man's dream," a source of fever and infection, and just as "medicine was philosophy at work," so was philosophy "medicine for the individual and for society." A French thinker speculated that legislators and judges would give way to physicians; while to Thomas Percival, the English hospital reformer, physicians were "strangers to superstition and enthusiasm [that is, fanaticism]" in the vanguard of the campaign for progress. In the view of Percival and many others, the doctor did more than simply cure disease, as though that weren't enough: he cured habits, reformed persons, and promoted the health of the body politic. Such an established figure was the reformer who speaks in the name of medicine that Flaubert satirizes the type in the person of Homais, the journalist-pharmacist and tireless campaigner for social hygiene, in *Madame Bovary.*

> "Despite the network of prejudices that still covers part of the map of Europe [writes Homais in an article for the *Rouen Beacon*], light is nevertheless beginning to penetrate our countryside. And so, last Tuesday, our small city of Yonville was the scene of a surgical experiment that is, at the same time, an act of great philanthropy. . . ."

The experiment costs the patient his leg. Almost in the manner of a Dickens character, Homais speaks like a repeating mechanism, and what he repeats are certain formulas of enlightenment.

Nor did the magnification of the physician's role limit itself to Europe. A chapter of Christopher Lasch's critical study of the forces converging on the American family is entitled, in irony, "Doctors to a Sick Society." Among the works there cited is *Society as the Patient: Essays on Culture and Personality.* By the mid-twentieth century, observes Lasch, progressive minds had become "highly receptive to medical modes of thought. Enlightened opinion now identified itself with the medicalization of society: the substitution of medical and psychiatric authority for the authority of parents, priests, and lawgivers." Did the bearers of enlightened opinion realize that in the name of innovation they were repeating terms and phrases laid down perhaps two hundred years before?

To *cure* ills is to do more than do something about them: it is to eradicate them, to destroy them at the source, an ambition that claims for itself the authority of science. Closely allied to the image of the reformer as physician to the world—a fixture in the publicity of reform—is the argument that publicity itself cures social ills. That is what Bentham had in mind when he wrote that "under the auspices of publicity, no evil can continue." Evil cannot continue because it has been cured. The public image of the reformer as physician and the claimed medicinal properties of publicity blend into each other. Both are in evidence in one of the most admired documents in the literature of reform.

So fixed is the notion of the physician to society that religion itself has been redefined, by some, as social medicine. Among the religious thinkers enlisted by those interested in "the medicalization of religion" are Martin Buber and Paul Tillich. Both are mentioned in Martin Luther King's famous "Letter from Birmingham Jail," a religious statement cast in the language of self-realization psychology but heightened with the imagery of medicine.

> Like a boil that can never be cured so long as it is covered up but must be opened with all its ugliness to the natural medicines of air and light, injustice must be exposed, with all the

tension its exposure creates, to the light of human conscience and the air of national opinion, before it can be cured.

Segregation, states King, is a "disease," the action of protesters an "antidote," the discontent of his people "healthy." Evidently Martin Luther King thought it possible to act as a sort of physician to millions. But perhaps it was possible to have this idea because so many others had had it and voiced it that it no longer seemed exorbitant. The cancer community, for its part, employs something very like the rhetoric of the "Letter from Birmingham Jail" in arguing that it is time for cancer to stop being a kind of ugly public secret, in demanding that it be put before the world in a way that cannot be ignored, in ascribing to publicity itself a saving power. By an accident of history, cancer has become tangled up with the rhetoric of liberation.

FROM Sissela Bok's belief that a doctor's rationale for lying "has to be capable of being made public," to the use of ribbons to raise awareness of cancer and gain the sympathy of society, to the belief that we have at last emerged from the dark ages when not all could be said or shown, publicity is considered a cure for ills and a force for human emancipation. Yet to be emancipated we must first have been in bondage. According to an influential way of thinking, to argue well is not so much to marshal evidence as to expose all that interferes with the reception of evidence in the first place—the prejudices that distort understanding, the "false consciousness" discoloring our entire mentality, the fears that hold us captive. It is to undo mental bondage. A lot of cancer rhetoric invests heavily in the familiar yet too little questioned theory that minds are enthralled to ignorance and fear, and that this thralldom, once exposed, is on the way to being broken. Much as our culture has cleared itself of the errors and delusions of the past, so does publicity break the spell of cancer and so does the patient overcome the shame, even the power, of cancer by going public. But, like the idea of the physician to a sick society, the image of publicity as a liberator finds a reception not because of its bold novelty but, on the contrary, because it has been so long in place. In *The Brothers Karamazov*, Dmitri's defense lawyer—himself a Clarence Darrow–like public figure—already speaks as a believer in the public exercise of reason as the best remedy for prejudice, cruelty, and backwardness. In so doing, however, even he sounds themes already traditional, at least in the West. At this point it may be fitting to look into some of the sources of the belief in publicity as a vehicle of enlightenment.

Traditionally, men of power claimed the right to display themselves in the most brilliant light. Not only was their code of honor aggressively theatrical and their conspicuous consumption a badge of privilege, but their power itself raised them above the unregarded and the ignoble into the light of public notice. At the same time power employed secrecy as an instrument of rule, cloaking itself in mystery, keeping its reasons to itself, denying the laity the right to judge political acts. The complement of the spectacle of power was the privilege of secrecy, the extreme example of this conjunction being the system of criminal justice prevailing in most of Europe before the age of the French Revolution: legal procedures carried out in secret, punishments carried out in public. In all probability the mystique of power owed more to the compound of theatrical display and concealed intentions and methods than to either one alone. In France the attack on ostentation overlapped with an attack on "the secrets of ministerial cabinets and royal councils." Not only in France, however, were both show and secrecy thrown into question. Around the time of the French Revolution, all aspects of the traditional formation came under challenge. State secrets were questioned, the ostentatious style of the elite anatomized and deplored, the nature of publicity itself investigated, and even habits of consumption revolutionized. Middle-class Britons engaged in conspicuous consumption of their own, and one of the inventors of modern salesmanship, Josiah Wedgwood, introduced such publicity devices as the showroom, the catalogue, and the guarantee, using the royalty of Europe as, in effect, celebrity endorsements for his wares.

Of all models of publicity, probably the most elevated is Kant's, its elevation corresponding to a certain lack of material content. In contrast to a twentieth-century regime claiming popular support, the state in Kant's Prussia drew a curtain between itself and a populace wholly excluded from political life. Behind this barrier it enjoyed the traditional privilege of secrecy—a tradition fraying in England, where the "secret" collusion of Parliament and crown was decried by many, as Kant himself did; and in France, where in 1775 the president of a high Parisian court issued a remonstrance urging the opening up of the political system to the light of publicity. The idealization of publicity is one index of the changing nature of the "bourgeois public sphere" at this time. Another is the challenge to traditionally privileged information like the size of the national debt, the content of parliamentary debates—more or less secret even in eighteenth-century America—or, as in France, the proceedings of judicial tribunals. "The principle of publicity was . . . held up in opposition to the practice of secrets of state," the former being identified with a community of literate, propertied men who spoke in the name of the general good. Committed to the free exercise of critical reason, offended by the paternalism that judges human beings incapable of self-rule, Kant himself affirms the right of citizens to speak in print on all public questions. Even such traditionally undiscussable matters of state as military policy and taxation are subject, he believes, to public debate. Publicity in this sense entails the critical discussion of issues of common concern—an idea still resonant in American life, which is only fitting, considering that Kant was influenced by the ideals of the American Revolution in the first place.

When Sissela Bok argues that a rationale for deceit has to stand the test of publicity, she writes in the tradition of Kant. According to Kant, right itself has a public quality. If moral action has the character of legislation, and if laws in turn need to be public if they are legitimately to *be* laws, then moral action must be consistent with being made public. An act that meets the test of public disclosure, that even requires disclosure to achieve its end, is a moral act. "When man was innocent and virtuous," writes Rousseau, "he liked to have the gods as witnesses to his actions." Kant settles for human witnesses, though for him too openness of heart is the proof of moral intention. In a world of kings where power claims the privilege of secrecy, where deceit is an element of rule, the Kantian demand of openness affirms the dawning capacity of citizens to rule themselves.

But if Kantian publicity challenges the secrecy in which power veils itself, it also rejects the visual brilliance of the aristocratic style. That is to say, it partakes of the abstract nature of reason in contrast to the theatricality of aristocratic display. With their elegant costumes and coaches, their generally opulent presentation of themselves, the aristocracy commanded a public attention that raised them above all those condemned to live and toil in obscurity—a theatrical grandeur, however, that increasingly appeared corrupt to critical minds. To Adam Smith, himself apparently an influence on Kant, it seemed that a craving for notice was both the driving motive of socioeconomic activity and the poisoner of moral values. In reply to the question of why men work so hard to imitate the rich, Smith answers that they want the *publicity* of the rich. "The man of rank and distinction . . . is observed by all the world. Every body is eager to look at him," whereas the poor are unregarded and despised. Though a defender of hierarchy, Smith makes it plain that he considers the hunger for public adulation "the great and most universal cause of the corruption of our moral sentiments." The man of power who presents himself for public worship is a corruption of Rousseau's innocent, so virtuous that he wants his actions surveyed by heaven.

As Smith explains, the rich possess a kind of visual charisma. The Kantian standard demotes the visual symbolism of aristocratic society in favor of a more abstract and rational form of publicity. If men are to put aside their "assigned role as an *audience* for the displays of power and exhibitions of art" staged by their rulers, if they are to go from the childlike status of political wards to the responsible status of citizens, they will have to learn the publicity of print. The Kantian ideal accordingly raises print over those theatrical representations that Rousseau, Kant's mentor, condemned so sharply. It was the importance of a free press that a contemporary of Kant had in mind when he wrote that "the law had no critics, morals had no supervisor, [and] reason was monopolized" until Providence said, "Let the human race become free! And publicity appeared." The appearance of such discourse in Germany suggests how generally

available, how public the language of the Enlightenment had become. In contrast to the corrupt publicity of luxury is the rational
publicity of the word.

Just as "the bourgeois public sphere of the cities, unlike the visually absorbed absolutist public sphere, was oriented around . . .
printed texts," so the Kantian norm of publicity envisions a group
of readers dispersed in space yet bound by common abstract principles. "A man of learning . . . may through his writings address a
public in the truest sense of the word," which is also to say that the
public of print is truer than the public of theater, held captive by the
aristocratic spectacle. Print does not appeal to the lust of the eye. To
revolutionaries in France, print was "the sign and guarantee of liberty," almost as if it warranted the honor of the goddess Liberty as
chastity warrants the honor of a woman. As print once broke the
grip of the Catholic church over Europe, so it would now break the
empire of priests and kings and put an end to the idolatry of error.
As readers belong to the abstract community of print, so citizens—
men in their public capacity—belong to the community of law.
One of the beauties of readers is that being spread out in space, they
do not have the intimacy of a conspiracy. A reading public does not
form cabals like those that obsessed the revolutionaries of France to
the point of mania, or factions like those so worrying to the framers
of the American Constitution. Not harboring secret designs, readers themselves can pass the Kantian test.

Kant wasn't the first to think of publicity as a check on the in-
defensible. In the politically charged atmosphere of prerevolutionary
France it was argued that the publication of trial briefs would clear
up the corruption endemic to a secret system of justice. Wrote one
lawyer: if you want to put a stop to iniquity, "threaten to unveil it,
to expose it to daylight in all of its ugliness." Often sensational in

their impact, such briefs appealed over the heads of the judicial authorities to the republic of print, which theoretically included all readers. It was in this tradition that Martin Luther King would expose the brutality of racism in all its ugliness, appealing over the heads of local magistrates to the court of national opinion (though for this very reason he must have seemed to his critics a mere publicity seeker). With their genius for marketing, the mass media have since cashed in the King principle, presenting every airing of a previously taboo issue, every breach of the threshold of reserve, as the fall of a Bastille. The continuing appeal of this rhetoric of boldness is one of the more ironic aftereffects of the French Revolution.

AS THOUGH to remind commoners that they had no right to stand out as public persons at all—that they were background and not figure—many punishments from the pillory to the gallows traditionally exposed the criminal to the eyes of the public. As some Englishmen argued in 1759, a merely private flogging does not offer the salutary example of a punishment in front of the crowd. It was during the lifetime of Kant that this form of publicity first came under heavy criticism, an attack that led eventually to the extinction of such spectacles in the West. Said Benjamin Rush in 1787,

> I can only hope that the time is not far away when gallows, pillory, scaffold, flogging and wheel will, in the history of punishment, be regarded as the marks of the barbarity of centuries and . . . proofs of the feeble influence of reason and religion over the human mind.

Some decades later, when a reformer argued in the English Parliament that "the printer and his types" promote good order better than "the gibbet and the hulks," it was as if one form of publicity were being advocated in another's place. A man of the Enlightenment and no champion of dark customs, Kant himself purifies the act of judgment, exposing "maxims" and not physical persons to public scrutiny—scrutiny no longer jeering but merely critical. Where the condemned had once been forced to publish their own guilt by the exhibition of their bodies, the Kantian citizen imagines the publication of his intentions to an abstract community of equals. Like a distant descendant of someone sentenced to the pillory or the stake, the citizen recoils in shame at the thought of exposing the moral ugliness of his maxims to the disapproving gaze of an abstract community. Some things are fit to be shown and seen because other things are not.

Almost from its inception, public opinion contained an element of opposition. Some of the inventors of modern publicity held no official position. Wedgwood was a provincial in a nation theoretically centered on London. A delicate problem he confronted in his approaches to Parliament on behalf of a manufacturers' lobby was how to avoid the appearance of political effrontery. If his group had "no legal existence," how could it claim a right to be heard at all? But neither did public opinion itself exist legally. The tribunal of opinion was situated outside established judicial and political institutions. More generally, all those moderns who draped themselves in classical costume as they sought to construct a public realm found in antiquity a source of validation outside standing institutions. The proudest construction of modernity, the public realm, in this sense rests on an act of imagination. And in part for that reason it was itself subject to change. It was in the alternative space opened up by the outsiders and insurgents and informal jurors of the reading public that the politically excluded later came to voice their claims. One of those who helped define the woman question, Mary Woll-stonecraft, used Kant's terms when she argued that women's self-incurred immaturity had to end: that the time had come for women to pass from subjects to citizens, from corrupt dependence to rational self-government.

Kant himself led an isolated life and held no political position. Other inventors of modern publicity, such as Rousseau and Bentham, stood outside the official public theater, apart from established positions of honor. Perhaps it only follows that for Bentham, too, publicity had an oppositional character. Indeed, whatever the philosophical differences between himself and Kant, he too envisioned publicity as a tribunal before which existing practices could be tried or tested. For Bentham, publicity is a kind of secular miracle, a natural and potent instrument of discipline far superior to old methods, a remedy of ills. Just as he aspired to play physician to millions, so in his view did publicity itself have a curative property. "Without publicity, no good is permanent: under the auspices of publicity, no evil can continue." But surely this is too pat. That no evil can withstand publicity (as though slavery had been a closely kept secret) is as doubtful as the claim that every human phenomenon masks a contrary reality. All in all, though, the right of opposition is still the best security against violations of what Kant and others called the rights of man, and in the age of the gulag and the death factory, of organized disappearances and induced famine, it performs a more urgent function than ever. While no kind of publicity can prevent all evils, the free expression of opposing views may at least prevent the worst evils.

In some respects, however, the Enlightenment ideal of publicity translates awkwardly into our own age. Those who would bring the most private things into the public realm, as if to do so were an act of emancipation, are interested not in shaming vice but in overcoming shame. In challenging darkness and silence, they borrow the rhetoric of the Enlightenment, transplanting it, however, from a world where the few ruled the many to one of representative government. Here then is another example of storming a fortress already deserted. One reason some of today's critics are so fond of the notion of conspiracy—conspiracies of silence and conspiratorial corporations—may be that only something as shadowy and baleful as a conspiracy can begin to account for dark silences without kings, priests, and other traditional enemies of enlightenment behind them. Conspiracies fill the absence of traditional oppressors. Ironically, though, just as the critics of silence repeat long-established arguments under the guise of innovation, so allegations of conspiracy repeat the countless claims of that kind during the age of the Enlightenment itself. Gordon Wood writes that "everywhere people sensed designs within designs, cabals within cabals: there were court conspiracies, backstairs conspiracies, ministerial conspiracies, factional conspiracies, . . . even conspiracies of gigantic secret societies that . . . spanned the Atlantic."

EVERYONE HAS a medical horror story. Mine concerns being suspected of conspiring, in essence, against the well-being of my daughter.

The birth of our first child was a day of great joy, joy I have carried somewhere within ever since. But while she was a healthy infant, she grew poorly and before long slipped beneath the first percentile of the growth chart. At the age of eighteen months she weighed perhaps eighteen pounds, and it was at that time that we three left for a year in the Bay Area, taking medical records with us.

Our daughter's pediatrician from birth (here Dr. Harrison) had seemed concerned but not alarmed over this too-small child, and that seemed about right, seeing that he himself was perhaps five foot two.

While seeking out another pediatrician in Berkeley, it occurred to me for some reason to look over the medical records. In them our child was described as a case of "failure to thrive"—phrasing that seemed all at once ominous, euphemistic, and peculiar, like a code word. Delving into the medical literature on failure to thrive, I found ambiguous insinuations, talk of the psychosocial deficiencies of the mother, suspicions of neglect and abuse. Children failing to thrive can be taken from their parents and placed in a hospital to be properly cared for. Convinced, perhaps, that every human phenomenon hides a contrary reality, or more likely just contaminated with all the publicity about child abuse, our pediatrician suspected that under the appearance of loving parents we were somehow starving our child. Enraged at the man's false imaginings and backhandedness (for he showed a friendly face while confiding his suspicions to the medical records), I wrote Dr. Harrison from Berkeley, disputing his diagnosis in the plainest terms. He replied by phone that when he used the term "failure to thrive," he didn't mean what other people meant, only that the cause of poor growth was unknown. As now seems clear, here was a man whose own modification of the tradition of the doctor to a sick society was the doctor as social worker. Really it wasn't much of a modification. Thomas Percival, writing at the turn of the nineteenth century, argued for a medical police force with the power to remove the infected poor from their homes and confine them in hospitals.

We returned from Berkeley when our child was not quite three.

Some twenty years later, as chance would have it, we found ourselves across the dinner table at a friend's house from a short, talkative man—Dr. Harrison. Though I knew better than to grenade the evening by identifying myself, I did make some remarks about our daughter thriving. What I wanted to say was, "She's as tall as you are!" I eyed him closely and caught no sign of recognition.

The next evening the phone rang. "I will never forget the misunderstanding we had over your daughter," said Dr. Harrison. "It was the worst incident in my professional life." With our daughter flourishing, the old dragon of anger had lost its fire, but even so there was going to be no meeting of the minds with Dr. Harrison. Over dinner the evening before he had mentioned that he was now seeing children suspected by the schools of being sexually abused. He said this facing—knowingly facing—two parents he had once suspected of denying food to their own child. It was like meeting Monsieur Homais in person. He was still bringing dark secrets to light, still exposing the cankers of a sick society.

We exchanged civilities and hung up.

THE PUBLIC AND THE PRIVATE

HARBORING A CANCER without symptoms and treated with radioactive iodine that also left no visible trace (in contrast to the ravages of other cancer treatments), I had the sense of leading a double life: one that presented itself to the eye and one known only to myself and a few others. Every day I crossed paths with many who would never discover the change that had taken place within me. Inset into the Middle English romance *Sir Gawain and the Green Knight* are wonderful scenes of the hero conversing in fine style even while his mind is oppressed with thoughts of his own impending execution. I acquired a new appreciation of Gawain's position. So covert is the disease that at times it recedes from awareness only to exert its presence all the same, like a stone you carry around in your shoe all day, ignored yet felt. Some weeks after surgery, when I ran into a vague acquaintance, it came out— how, I can't say, since these are things spoken of with reluctance— that he was having medical problems, prostate problems. All at once we were members of one secret society of the body. For me cancer has been a matter of secrecy, an education in the covert, and if only for that reason the publicity of cancer sounds false to my ears.

[*183*]

Certainly the private and the public are different realms, different frames of reference. The distinction between the two is etched into the beginnings of our literature, the *Odyssey* differing from the *Iliad* in treating the private side of existence. Thus, for example, Homer's portrayal of Odysseus in solitude and privation; thus the prominence of women in the poem, and, closely related, its focus on the household. The private and the public: these terms and categories remain with us, even as publicity—the shimmer that hovers above our way of life like a mirage—brings word of the world into our private dwellings and brings private things to public view, even to the showing of birth on television.

How strange to learn that François Mitterand, the president of France, suffered through prostate cancer all his years in office until at last he was incapacitated. How strange it must have been for Boswell, paying a visit to Rousseau in his retreat, to find the sage in a kaftan owing to a urinary ailment. Bidding his enlightened mentor good-bye on December 5, 1764, Boswell added, "But I shall come back." Said Rousseau, "I don't promise to see you. I am in pain. I need a chamber-pot every minute."

BEFORE MONTAIGNE, no one had ever written to the world about the experience of kidney stones.

> The fear and pity felt by people for this illness gives you something to glory about. . . . There is pleasure in hearing them say about you: "There's fortitude for you! There's long-suffering!" They see you sweating under the strain, turning pale, flushing, trembling, sicking up everything including blood, suffering curious spasms and convulsions, sometimes shedding huge

tears from your eyes, excreting frightening kinds of urine. . . . You, meanwhile, chat with those about you, keeping your usual expression, occasionally clowning with your servants, defending your corner in a tense argument, apologizing for any sign of pain and understating your suffering.

Even the essay "On Experience," the source of this passage, is rich with classical maxims and verses. More than mere adornments, these are also the anchorages of Montaigne's thought, a sort of remedy against his own mutability. Even as he creates a new register of introspection and opens new ranges of expression, Montaigne uses and honors the public language of learning. When Rousseau proclaims that he is about to reveal himself as no one has ever done before, he upstages Montaigne and promises, in effect, to turn from the world of books to the direct utterances of the heart. Nor, for all of his originality, does Montaigne ever imply that by breaking with the past and speaking of himself as none had ever spoken he was somehow freeing others from the yoke of tradition.

In our time, freeing others from the yoke of tradition has become a fixed pose, a convention, even, strangely, a tradition. Defying taboos and portraying the past as a long night of repression, liberators use arguments and strike attitudes that for a long while have been the very currency of opposition. Presenting themselves as breakers of molds, they deal almost obsessively in ready-made ideas. Among these is the imperative of transparency. As though the health of the body politic demanded the exposure of all things concealed just as the practice of medicine makes visible the interior of the body, many today seem to wish for the abolition of concealment— a world of glass. My sense is that when the most private experiences of human life are held up as public examples, they are falsified precisely in being placed in the standard categories and styles that dominate the public realm.

The Death of Ivan Ilych opens with an illustration of this effect. In a newspaper "still damp from the press," the dead man's colleagues come across his death notice:

> Surrounded by a black border were the words: "Praskovya Fedorovna Golovina, with profound sorrow, informs relatives and friends of the demise of her beloved husband Ivan Ilych Golovin, Member of the Court of Justice, which occurred on February 4th of this year 1882."

Like the black border itself, the words "profound" and "beloved" are at once conventional public expressions of mourning, giveaways, and examples of the fatal hypocrisy to which the hero lost his life. Transposed into an acceptably public idiom, the story of Ivan Ilych's life and death loses its truth altogether. (In dramatizing her own sorrow and suffering, Praskovya Fedorovna also adopts a public style: that of the playhouse. With Ivan Ilych on his deathbed, she goes to see Sarah Bernhardt.) Probably Tolstoy would consider opinion polls no more accurate registers of truth than the obituary that sets the tone for *The Death of Ivan Ilych*.

In part, Tolstoy wrote *War and Peace* to correct a similar falsification. Just after a battle—before they discover the official version of the event and square their memories and impressions with it—soldiers will honestly report their experience. Soon enough, however, falsehood sets in.

> Make a round of the troops immediately after a battle . . . and ask any of the soldiers and senior and junior officers how the affair went: you will be told what all these men experienced

and saw, and you will form a majestic, complex, infinitely varied, depressing and indistinct impression. . . . Two or three days later the reports begin to be handed in. Talkers begin to narrate how things happened which they did not see; finally a general report is drawn up, and on this report the general opinion of the army is formed. Everyone is glad to exchange his own doubts and questionings for this deceptive, but clear and always flattering presentation.

It is because Tolstoy suspected the neatness of narrative that *War and Peace* itself defies every tradition of narrative unity. The reader of *War and Peace* "hesitates frequently because the book includes numerous events and characters that may have either great consequence or no consequence at all. In Tolstoy's book, both possibilities are always present, as they are in life." One with prostate cancer becomes keenly aware of the Tolstoyan alternatives, the disease itself being capable of turning lethal or lying inert—as though it had been sent to mock the pride of human knowledge.

WHEN THE EXPERIENCE of cancer is stylized and made the subject of publicity campaigns, when cancer develops its own myths, emblems, verbal formulas, and even product line, falsity enters in, much as Tolstoy's soldiers falsify their own experience in fitting it to the official, public line. According to the heroic rhetoric now in fashion, cancer patients are themselves soldiers to be honored for battling the disease and indeed battling shame—as though these history-scarred words had at last found their proper use. Whatever the results of the War on Cancer declared by President Nixon, the rhetoric of conquest and the vision of cancer as an invader have contributed to a redefinition of patient as agent and victim as hero.

Perhaps my attention is caught by the symbols, myths, and rhetoric of cancer because these things are the stuff of literature. Literature also has a lot to say about the insufficiency of standard categories and verbal formulas. As a force that runs through different categories of literature itself—prose and verse, narrative and drama, tragedy and comedy, and probably any others that come to mind—satire in particular breaks through the codified, the fixed, the frozen. We might say the experience of cancer satirizes the public conventions of the disease. Satire springs from

> the feeling that experience is bigger than any set of beliefs about it. The satirist demonstrates the infinite variety of what men do by showing the futility, not only of saying what they ought to do, but even of attempts to systematize or formulate a coherent scheme of what they do.

Thus the many visions of marriage, from romantic felicity to life-long humiliation, in *Pride and Prejudice,* a satiric investigation of failings curable and incurable. But thus too the essays in *War and Peace,* with their argument of futility and their tone of demonstration. A perfect satiric example of systematic coherence would be the syllogism Ivan Ilych learned in school, which made no impression and did no good:

> The syllogism he had learnt from Kiesewetter's Logic: "Caius is a man, men are mortal, therefore Caius is mortal," had always seemed to him correct as applied to Caius, but it certainly didn't apply to himself.

In keeping with satire's accommodation of variety—reminiscent of the "infinite variety" of the original reports from the field—both *The Brothers Karamazov* and *The Death of Ivan Ilych* are strongly satiric works in spite of their authors being virtual opposites.

In *The Brothers Karamazov* a distortion effect sets in as Dmitri's trial becomes a public spectacle, and indeed as soon as the case finds its way into the hands of public officers at all. Like someone filling in a form, the interrogation team simply fills in the details of a crime whose outline they think they already know. In the course of Dmitri's questioning by these men committed to the idea of his guilt and prepossessed of a theory of the crime, one brings up a recent case where a thief sewed money in the piping of his cap. They sequester Dmitri's cap. In and of itself, this little action constitutes a satiric parable of the power of ready-made ideas and theoretical systems. As a character, Dmitri Karamazov is himself bigger than everything said about him.

A satiric counterpart of the physician who enriches himself at the expense of those in suffering (like the greedy pretender who looks in on the family of Captain Snegiryov in *The Brothers Karamazov*) is the patient who only imagines himself sick in the first place, the fool of his own habit of pretending. Deceived in one case, the patient is self-deceived in the other. After pretending for decades to be sick, the legendary Mrs. Churchill of *Emma* at last proves her point by dying, an event that restores her reputation and clears her "of all the fancifulness, and all the selfishness of imaginary complaints." In our own health-crazed culture, where the commercials on the evening news range from one class of drugs to another, and where not only new drugs but new conditions are invented, a lot of work seems to go into confusing the distinction between valid and fictive ailments. Beyond what the economist and the satirist once called imaginary wants lie imaginary conditions and imaginary cures. Accordingly, as if some vast new China market had been discovered in our own midst, pills, therapies, tonics, potions, and advice are sold aggressively and sold everywhere. Along with the pursuit of well-being goes the cultivation of anxiety and discontent and the medicalization of potentially everything. The more anxious our concerns, the more publicity they generate, publicity which in turn authorizes ailments and makes them distinctly fashionable. "Social phobia, all but invisible until the 1990s, now appears to affect the population in such epidemic proportion that the launch of Paxil as an anti-shyness agent was a media event."

But if we can deceive ourselves into being sick, can we not also deceive ourselves into being well?

It was Dmitri Karamazov's folly to believe that he could escape with Grushenka, the object of his infatuation, to a new and virtuous life at the same time he was incriminating himself by word and deed in the eyes of the world. It was Ivan Karamazov's folly to believe that he could walk away from his household at the very moment he implicated himself, however ambiguously, in his father's murder. Much of the comedy and tragedy of *The Brothers Karamazov* lies in the author's treatment of these quixotic illusions of escape. The theme of disentanglement and escape is written into the tale of Ivan Ilych too, and not only in his wife and daughter's flight to the theater while he lies on his deathbed. In a moment of dark comedy, the widow of Ivan Ilych catches her mourning shawl on the edge of a table.

> Peter Ivanovich rose to detach it, and the springs of the pouffe, relieved of his weight, rose also and gave him a push. The

widow began detaching the shawl herself, and Peter Ivanovich again sat down. . . . But the widow had not quite freed herself and Peter Ivanovich got up again, and again the pouffe rebelled and even creaked.

Just such a mishap as here befalls his wife brings on Ivan Ilych's illness. And he too tries to get free. Just as Ivan Ilych seeks to escape from his wife only to return of necessity to her vulgarity and her grievances, so too does he seek to escape his disease only to find himself again in its power. Whether it will be so with me I do not know, though I do recall imagining myself free of cancer when in fact I was primed for it.

RECENTLY, in looking over an article clipped from a June 1999 issue of the *New Republic,* I was astonished to find that there on one of its pages, plain as a billboard, stands an ad reading in part:

ATTENTION

PROSTATE

CANCER

PATIENTS

Before you have radical
surgery, know that
TheraSeed may be
a better choice—an
outpatient treatment
that's easier on you.

Though my eyes must have run over these words, I have no memory of them. They never registered. Still some months from a

biopsy, I had never heard of titanium seeds and had no thought of prostate cancer. Besides, who dwells on advertisements? If Ivan Ilych only later recognized the bruise to his side as the onset of his decline, so only now, in retrospect, do I perceive this ad's pertinence to my own case—in fact, perceive it at all. I suspect that even as my eyes brushed over the words "prostate cancer," the disease had already taken root, too deep for perception, a black illustration of the principle that what is important cannot be noticed. Or rather, even as I supposed that a person either had cancer or not, and that I did not, the precursors of cancer were already present, soon to wake up from their long dormancy.

A STONE WITHOUT A CHERRY

"WHY NOT BE a Johnny Appleseed for Prostate Cancer? Order pins to spread in your community to raise Prostate Cancer awareness." I think of seeds, seeds, Manna like coriander seed, the seed of Onan, the mustard seed of faith, Brueghel's plowman, a packet of beans. Tall oaks from little acorns grow. "Softly she gave me in my mouth the seedcake warm and chewed," says Bloom to himself, his story itself seeded with references to Odysseus, son of Laertes and seed of Zeus. "Consider your seed," says Dante's Ulysses to his men. Deep in Ivan Ilych lies the seed of tragic capacity. Dmitri Karamazov reaps what he sows and then some. The capitalist world, they say, bears within itself the seeds of its own destruction. "That the root, stem, leaves, petals, &c. of this crocus cohere to one plant, is owing to an antecedent Power or Principle in the Seed."

So difficult to distinguish are good and evil, says Milton, that "those confused seeds which were imposed on Psyche as an incessant labor to cull out and sort asunder were not more intermixed." Seeds innumerable. Seeds of metal numbering exactly 103, the shrapnel of healing, tiny metal hyphens shown for size against a penny. Seeds that kill growth, that produce no rain but a cloud, a radioactive cloud. "A pregnant woman can greet you briefly and then move to a distance six or more feet away." During the first half-life, while I was still a hazard, our first grandchild was born. Half-life and new life.

Cancer itself seems to germinate, lying latent for ten, twenty, forty years, slowly accumulating its lethal factors, growing as if from seed. "One event always flows uninterruptedly from another."

You hear of trees that wait for fire to release their seeds. Can cancer cells ride out the fire of radiation, awaiting their time? I am left with a seed of doubt.

NOTES

Preface: Cancer and Cant

p. xi, corpses dust: Paul Fussell, *The Great War and Modern Memory* (Oxford: Oxford University Press, 1975), p. 22.

p. xi, "devour the weak": Cited in Walter Houghton, *The Victorian Frame of Mind* (New Haven: Yale University Press, 1957), p. 320.

p. xii, "our fallen soldiers": Barbara Ehrenreich, "Welcome to Cancerland," *Harper's*, November 2001.

p. xii, shot down over North Vietnam: Rep. Randy (Duke) Cunningham, R-Calif., *Minneapolis Star-Tribune*, April 14, 2002.

p. xii, "genuine healing will not have occurred": Jeremy Geffen, M.D., cited in *New York Times* online, April 23, 2002.

p. xiv, "the flick of an intention": Deepak Chopra, *Perfect Health: The Complete Mind Body Guide* (New York: Random House, 1991; 2000), p. 16.

p. xiv, "not without dust and heat": John Milton, "Areopagitica."

p. xvi, "I have my own": Drs. Bill and Susie Buchholz, *Live Longer, Live Larger: A Holistic Approach for Cancer Patients and Families* (Sebastopol, Calif.: O'Reilly, 2001), p. 232.

p. xvii, "and think of what cannot be true": J. D. McClatchy, "Cancer," *Literary Imagination* 4.2 (2002): 264.

Polls, Statistics, Forms

p. 3, "effort to postpone death": Sissela Bok, *Lying: Moral Choice in Public and Private Life* (New York: Vintage, 1979), p. 233.

p. 4, "a threat to everyone": Kant, "Perpetual Peace," in *Political Writings,* tr. H. B. Nisbet (Cambridge, England: Cambridge University Press, 1992), p. 126.

p. 4, a game of pretend. In the classroom I have found teenagers especially bold to know the worst. Eighty percent is too low a figure.

p. 5, "speculation or hypothesis": Karl Mannheim, *Essays on Sociology and Social Psychology* (London: Routledge and Kegan Paul, 1953), p. 103.

p. 6, said yes: Robert M. Veatch, *Death, Dying, and the Biological Revolution* (New Haven: Yale University Press, 1989), p. 183.

p. 6, a condition potentially just that: Survey released by the National Prostate Cancer Campaign, July 24, 2001.

p. 7, "the period of contemplation": Fyodor Dostoevsky, *The Brothers Karamazov,* tr. Constance Garnett (New York: Viking, 1955), p. 150.

p. 7, "such important cumulative results": Iris Murdoch, *The Sovereignty of Good* (London: Routledge, 1970; 2001), p. 42.

p. 9, "into the courthouse": Dr. Richard N. Atkins in *San Francisco Chronicle,* March 26, 2002.

p. 9, "alternative for professional medical care": Buchholz, *Live Longer, Live Larger,* p. ii.

p. 12, "what manner of men they are that do it": John Stuart Mill, *On Liberty* (New York: Norton, 1975), p. 56.

p. 14, "towards an accused person": Leo Tolstoy, *Short Fiction,* tr. Michael R. Katz (New York: Norton, 1991), p. 142.

p. 14, reactions to cancer: David G. Bostwick, M.D., Gregory T. MacLennan, M.D., and Thayne R. Larson, M.D., *Prostate Cancer: What Every Man—and His Family—Needs to Know* (New York: Villard, 1996), p. 77.

p. 15, "would never come near us": *The Portable Tolstoy,* ed. John Bayley; tr. Aylmer and Louise Maude (New York: Viking Penguin, 1978), pp. 557–558.

p. 17 , says Tolstoy in *War and Peace:* Leo Tolstoy, *War and Peace,* tr. Aylmer and Louise Maude (Oxford: Oxford University Press, 1991), p. 880.

p. 17, the course of the game. Cf. Murdoch, *Sovereignty of Good,* p. 36.

p. 19, "virtually complete": Veatch, *Death, Dying, and the Biological Revolution,* p. 184.

p. 22, "will follow naturally": Murdoch, *Sovereignty of Good,* pp. 40–41.

p. 22, the ordinary politics of accusation: The organization is Breast Cancer Action.

p. 22, sincerity in modern philosophy: Murdoch, *Sovereignty of Good,* pp. 46, 48.

The Faithful Plowman

p. 24, "suffering humanity": Tolstoy, *War and Peace,* p. 1182.

p. 26, "extreme moments which 'ordinary life' covers over": Michael André Bernstein, *New Republic,* September 27, 1999.

p. 27, "the mill-horse round": Mill, *On Liberty* p. 104.

p. 28, "unsettled in the extreme": Jane Austen, *Complete Novels* (New York: Modern Library, n.d.), p. 464.

p. 28, "rise to distinction": Austen, *Complete Novels,* p. 598.

p. 28, "what is noticed *cannot* be important": Gary Saul Morson, *Hidden in Plain View: Narrative and Creative Potentials in 'War and Peace'* (Stanford: Stanford University Press, 1987), p. 130.

p. 28, where importance lies. In that Leopold Bloom does not recognize that he is undergoing the adventures of Odysseus, something like the irony of Brueghel's *Landscape* fills *Ulysses.*

p. 28, "without ever overemphasizing its importance": Mikhail Bakhtin, *The Dialogic Imagination,* tr. Caryl Emerson and Michael Holquist (Austin: University of Texas Press, 1981), pp. 193–194.

p. 30, "the peace of the mountains": George Steiner, *Tolstoy or Dostoevsky* (New Haven: Yale University Press, 1996), p. 82. On this page Steiner also refers to "Brueghel's Icarus plummeting into the calm sea as the ploughman walks his furrow in the foreground."

p. 30, "the joy of life": Tolstoy, *Short Fiction,* p. 152.

p. 31, forbidden knowledge: See Roger Shattuck, *Forbidden Knowledge: From Prometheus to Pornography* (San Diego: Harcourt Brace, 1996).

p. 31, "embraces every sort of variety": Michel de Montaigne, *The Essays, A Selection,* tr. M. A. Screech (Harmondsworth, Middlesex: Penguin, 1993), p. 391.

p. 33, "their human dignity": Primo Levi, *The Drowned and the Saved,* tr. Raymond Rosenthal (New York: Summit, 1988), p. 122.

Beyond Shame and Guilt

p. 34, Viagra is advised after surgery. But it is one thing, I realized, to receive this sort of advice in the doctor's office and another to nag, beg, or hint for Viagra at the prodding of commercials aimed at a national market.

p. 35, "I can help somebody get diagnosed earlier": Bostwick, MacLennan, and Larson, *Prostate Cancer,* p. 164. "Recognize and Manage Your Emotions": p. 76.

p. 35, "a wild leap of the will": Murdoch, *Sovereignty of Good,* p. 26.

p. 36, a lack of self-restraint: Susan Sontag, "AIDS and Its Metaphors," *New York Review of Books,* October 27, 1988.

p. 36, "their significance and emotional vibrancy": Rochelle Gurstein, *The Repeal of Reticence* (New York: Hill and Wang, 1996), p. 43.

p. 37, the baseless nature of guilt itself. Robert Jay Lifton once reported to me a comment by Hannah Arendt regarding his book on the Hiroshima survivors. "Excellent book, Dr. Lifton. But on one point you are wrong. There is no such thing as survivor guilt." According to Arendt, "It is only in a metaphorical sense that we can say we feel guilty for the sins of our fathers or of our people or of mankind, i.e., for deeds and misdeeds we have not done. Morally speaking, it is as wrong to feel guilty without having done something specific as it is to feel free of all guilt if one actually is guilty of something." "Personal Responsibility Under Dictatorship," *The Listener,* August 6, 1964, p. 185.

p. 40, "24-hour-a-day, seven-day-a-week effort": Testimony to the U.S. Senate Subcommittee on Labor, Health, & Human Services and Education Appropriations, June 16, 1999; reprinted at <www.mikemilken.com>.

p. 42, "had not been subject to criminal prosecution": "Mike Milken's Biography" at <www.mikemilken.com>.

p. 43, "I have never been motivated by money in my entire life": *Fortune,* September 30, 1996.

p. 44, changing oneself by changing one's habits: Charles Taylor, *Sources of the Self: The Making of the Modern Identity* (Cambridge, Mass.: Harvard University Press, 1989), p. 159.

The Breast and the Prostate

p. 47, "amongst the most malignant and clinically intransigent" forms of the disease: Mel Greaves, *Cancer: The Evolutionary Legacy* (Oxford: Oxford University Press, 2001), p. 83.

p. 47, "die *with,* not *of*": Shannon Brownlee, *New Republic,* April 22, 2002.

p. 48, "approximately the same number of lives": Milken testimony, June 16, 1999.

p. 48, "told to wait—for another disease": Cited in *Maclean's,* April 1, 2002.

p. 49, "women will continue to die from neglect of this disease": Barbara A. Brenner in BCA (Breast Cancer Action) Newsletter #31, August 1995.

p. 50, "a striking resemblance to the mall": Ehrenreich, "Welcome to Cancerland."

p. 51, "gifts of Matchbox cars." But don't Viagra ads try to get men to get their doctors to write prescriptions, by analogy with toy ads that get children to get their parents to open their wallets?

p. 54, "more disability and economic disadvantage than any other disorder": David Healy, "Good Science of Good Business?" *Hastings Center Report* 30, no. 2 (2000): 20.

p. 55, "if all women had their breasts removed at age 50": A statistician, Bradley Efron, cited in *New York Times* online, April 9, 2002.

p. 55, "manages their principal concerns": Alexis de Tocqueville, *Democracy in America,* Vol. 2, tr. Henry Reeve, Francis Bowen, Phillips Bradley (New York: Vintage, 1945), p. 336.

p. 56, "the panacea for all that they thought evil": Isaiah Berlin, *Four Essays on Liberty* (London: Oxford University Press, 1969), p. 177.

p. 56, the culture of health complaints: Robert Hughes, *Culture of Complaint* (New York: Warner, 1994).

p. 56, "Those who do not complain are never pitied": Austen, *Complete Novels,* p. 300.

p. 58, "the menials who, all this time, have been doing our dirty work": Richard Rorty, *Contingency, Irony, and Solidarity* (Cambridge, England: Cambridge University Press, 1989), p. 196.

Conspiracy of Silence

p. 60, "She was not to know": Tillie Olsen, *Tell Me a Riddle* (New York: Dell, 1961), p.86.

p. 62, "the first quarter of the twentieth century": Gurstein, *Repeal of Reticence,* p. 91.

p. 62, the very fruition of his own technique. On Bernays, see Stewart Justman, *The Psychological Mystique* (Evanston: Northwestern University Press, 1998).

p. 63, "transcendent, critical notions": Herbert Marcuse, *One-Dimensional Man* (Boston: Beacon Press, 1964), p. 85.

p. 64, "the contempt we have shown for her lessons": Jean-Jacques Rousseau, *A Discourse on Inequality*, tr. Maurice Cranston (Harmondsworth, Middlesex: Penguin, 1984), p. 149. Living rightly, the Houyhnhnms in *Gulliver's Travels* have no diseases.

p. 64, "the man I shall portray will be myself": Jean-Jacques Rousseau, *The Confessions*, tr. J. M. Cohen (Harmondsworth, Middlesex: Penguin, 1953), p. 17.

p. 64, "can hide nothing of what goes on inside": Cited in Jean Starobinski, *Jean-Jacques Rousseau: Transparency and Obstruction*, tr. Arthur Goldhammer (Chicago: University of Chicago Press, 1988), p. 254.

p. 65, "triumph over the machinations of men": Rousseau, *Confessions*, p. 525.

p. 65, "medical missteps and unfair allegations": Ehrenreich, "Welcome to Cancerland."

p. 65, "the cruelest possible persecution": Starobinski, *Transparency and Obstruction*, p. 244.

p. 66, "mystery and evil are almost synonymous": Starobinski, *Transparency and Obstruction*, p. 66.

p. 66, a Rousseauvian world. As when activist women "directly" exchanged stories of their experience.

p. 67, "racialized class patriarchal power": Zillah Eisenstein, *Manmade Breast Cancers* (Ithaca: Cornell University Press, 2001), p. 56.

p. 67, "a global capitalist patriarchal economy": Eisenstein, *Manmade Breast Cancers*, p. 173.

p. 67, "unsilencing": Eisenstein, *Manmade Breast Cancers*, p. 79.

p. 67, "became normal, necessary, and rational": Gordon S. Wood, "Conspiracy and the Paranoid Style: Causality and Deceit in the Eighteenth Century," *William and Mary Quarterly*, Third Series, 39 (1982): 417, 421. Zillah Eisenstein in *Manmade Breast Cancers* makes a show of rejecting simplistic notions of causality even as she trades on such notions, endorses the claim that 80 percent of all cancers result from "human produced carcinogens" (p. 73), and, like a conspiracy theorist, shows all things as being connected.

p. 68, "predict and control not only nature but [their] own society": Wood, "Conspiracy and the Paranoid Style," p. 413.

p. 68, the effects of the body's own hormones on the breast: Greaves, *Cancer*, p. 158.

p. 68, "to educate men about the disease": Bostwick, MacLennan, and Larson, *Prostate Cancer*, p. viii.

p. 69, "doctors do not know which one is most effective": *New York Times,* May 9, 2000.

p. 69, "information needs of primary care clinicians and of the public": <www.cdc.gov/cancer/prostate/index.htm>.

p. 70, "saying as little and meaning as much as possible": Northrop Frye, *Anatomy of Criticism* (New York: Atheneum, 1967), p. 40.

p. 70, a preference for the traditional institution of literature over its offshoot, journalism. On Austen, satire, and literature, see Stewart Justman, *The Springs of Liberty: The Satiric Tradition and Freedom of Speech* (Evanston: Northwestern University Press, 1999).

p. 70, nothing and no one of any interest is ever explicit: Gerald Bruns, *Inventions: Writing, Textuality, and Understanding in Literary History* (New Haven: Yale University Press, 1982), p. 115.

p. 70, "Let us have the luxury of silence": Austen, *Complete Novels,* p. 639.

p. 71, "which the great novelists fully realize but do not verbalize": George Steiner, *On Difficulty and Other Essays* (Oxford: Oxford University Press, 1978), p. 133.

p. 71, "Speech reaches into silence": Denis Donoghue speaking on "The Arts Without Mystery" in Missoula, Mont., April 22, 2002.

p. 71, "he never spoke in public": Bruns, *Inventions,* p. 40.

p. 72, "but always over *whole points of view*": M. M. Bakhtin, *Problems of Dostoevsky's Poetics,* tr. Caryl Emerson (Minneapolis: University of Minnesota Press, 1984), p. 96.

p. 73, "a humbler, gentler guy": *San Francisco Chronicle,* February 14, 2002; originally in *New York Times.*

Self and Others

p. 75, "accept death proudly and serenely like a god": Dostoevsky, *The Brothers Karamazov,* p. 789.

p. 76, "until one meets the desired specifications": Taylor, *Sources of the Self,* pp. 159–160.

p. 77, "to help you enjoy the pleasure of food": Introduction by Michael Milken to *The Taste for Living* by Beth Ginsberg; reprinted at <www.mikemilken.com>.

p. 79, "the right decision—right for you": Bostwick, MacLennan, and Larson, *Prostate Cancer,* pp. 94, 134.

p. 79, "the most torment of all": Tolstoy, *Short Fiction*, p. 166.

p. 80, "the charm of the social affections": David Hume, *Essays Moral, Political, and Literary* (Indianapolis: Liberty Classics, 1987), p. 151.

p. 80, "as easily and cheerfully as my best friends could desire": Letter from Adam Smith to William Strahan, in Hume, *Essays*, p. xliv.

p. 82, "internalize the urge and slay themselves": Bucholz, *Live Longer, Live Larger*, p. 332. The authors cite Carol Pearson, author of *The Hero Within*.

p. 82, "duality and equivocality and doubt": Hannah Arendt, *Totalitarianism*; Part 3 of *The Origins of Totalitarianism* (New York; Harcourt, Brace & World, 1968), p. 174.

p. 82, till death do us part. I was surprised to see the same figure used by Anatole Broyard in *Intoxicated by My Illness* (New York: Fawcett Columbine, 1992), p. 53. What is it about the bond between a man and a urologist that suggests a marriage?

p. 84, "whereof he knew nothing": John Locke, *Essays Concerning Human Understanding, Works*, Vol. II (London, 1823; Scientia Verlag Aalen, 1963), p. 64.

Compassion

p. 85, "tremble and shudder at the thought of what he feels": Adam Smith, *The Theory of Moral Sentiments* (Indianapolis: Liberty Classics, 1982), p. 9. Cf. Dr. Johnson in Rambler No. 60: "All joy or sorrow for the happiness or calamities of others is produced by an act of the imagination, that realizes the event, however fictitious, or approximates it, however remote, by placing us, for a time, in the condition of him whose fortunes we contemplate."

p. 86, "'How good how simple!' he thought": Tolstoy, *Short Fiction*, pp. 166–167.

p. 89, "would the mention of his name affect you": Herman Melville, *Selected Tales and Poems* (New York: Holt, Rinehart and Winston, 1950), p. 21.

History's Children

p. 92, "impose his self-righteous morality upon others": Gurstein, *Repeal of Reticence*, p. 129.

p. 93, "bewitchment and error": Taylor, *Sources of the Self*, p. 163.

p. 93, "right through to today": Taylor, *Sources of the Self*, p. 174.

p. 93, "beyond which life triumphs and continues": M. M. Bakhtin, *The Dialogic Imagination*, tr. Caryl Emerson and Michael Holquist (Austin: University of Texas Press, 1981), p. 193.

p. 93, "free from established custom": Taylor, *Sources of the Self,* p. 167.

p. 94, "We must learn to suffer whatever we cannot avoid": Michel de Montaigne, *The Essays: A Selection,* tr. M. A. Screech (Harmondsworth, Middlesex: Penguin, 1993), pp. 393–394.

p. 94, "good for the immune system": Breast Cancer Action Newsletter #71, May/June 2002.

Belief and Disbelief

p. 95, "irritating them instead of quietening them down": Montaigne, p. 392.

p. 96, "firmly entrenched": Lionel Trilling, *Sincerity and Authenticity* (Cambridge, Mass.: Harvard University Press, 1972), p. 142.

p. 98, "crawling out from underneath": *New York Times Book Review,* May 25, 1997.

p. 99, as one medical commentator surmises: Bob Arnot, *The Prostate Cancer Protection Plan* (Boston: Little, Brown, 2000), p. 28.

p. 99, "a half-baked Rousseauism": Northrop Frye, *The Well-Tempered Critic* (Bloomington: Indiana University Press, 1963), p. 42.

p. 100, "*Everything backfires*": Albert O. Hirschman, *The Rhetoric of Reaction* (Cambridge, Mass.: Harvard University Press, 1991), p. 12.

p. 101, "survived significantly longer than women who didn't attend": Bostwick, MacLennan, and Larson, *Prostate Cancer,* pp. 238–239.

p. 103, between the extremes of conventional and alternative medicine: Buchholz, *Live Longer, Live Larger,* pp. 278, 282, 22, 21.

p. 103, enhance the immune system: Bostwick, MacLennan, and Larson, *Prostate Cancer,* pp. 235, 239.

p. 104, "affect the course of history and events and even one's own health": Michael Milken as quoted in *Fortune,* September 30, 1996.

p. 104, following the seed treatment: *New Yorker,* May 29, 2001.

p. 106, "This is true for prostate cancer": Greaves, *Cancer,* p. 240.

The Will to Transparency: Jeremy Bentham

p. 108, "forcibly bringing it to light": Trilling, *Sincerity and Authenticity*, p. 142.

p. 109, say or even think: *Mill's Essays on Literature and Society*, ed. J. B. Schneewind (New York: Collier Books, 1965), p. 242.

p. 110, "a language familiar to everyone": Jeremy Bentham, *Works*, ed. John Bowring (New York: Russell and Russell, 1962), III, 209.

p. 110, "instead of using it as a piece of machinery": Broyard, *Intoxicated by My Illness*, p. 44.

p. 110, "was reserved for this . . . latter era": Thomas Carlyle, *Sartor Resartus*, in *Selections from the Writings of Thomas Carlyle*, ed. G. B. Tennyson (New York: Modern Library, 1969), p. 276.

p. 111, rather than the vernacular: Jürgen Habermas, *The Structural Transformation of the Public Sphere: An Inquiry into a Category of Bourgeois Society*, trs. Thomas Burger and Frederick Lawrence (Cambridge, Mass.: MIT Press, 1991), p. 9.

p. 111, icon by abstraction, theater by print: Sarah Maza, *Private Lives and Public Affairs: The Causes Célèbres of Prerevolutionary France* (Berkeley: University of California Press, 1993), p. 85.

p. 111, "the greatest degree of *transparency*, and thence of simplicity, possible": Bentham, *Works*, IX, 203.

p. 112, "concealment and yet revelation": Carlyle, *Sartor Resartus*, p. 276.

p. 112, "to regain the transparency we have lost": Starobinski, *Transparency and Obstruction*, p. 12.

p. 112, "if we do not dread being seen": Bentham, *Works*, II, 310.

p. 113, "not to infection and degradation": Cited in Christopher Lasch, *Haven in a Heartless World: The Family Besieged* (New York: Basic Books, 1979), p. 15.

p. 113, "training the rising race in the path of education": Bentham, *Works*, IV, 40.

p. 113, a name for naiveté among their opponents. On the hyperbolic claims of self-promoters in the age of the printing press, see Elizabeth Eisenstein, *The Printing Revolution in Early Modern Europe* (Cambridge, England: Cambridge University Press, 1993), p. 142: "The same publicity system that enabled instrument makers to advertise their wares and contribute to public knowledge also encouraged an output of more sensational claims. Discoveries of philosophers' stones, the keys to all knowledge, the cures to all ills were proclaimed by self-taught and self-professed miracle workers who often proved more adept at press agentry than at any of the older arts."

p. 114, the last public gestures of the condemned: Michel Foucault, *Discipline and Punish: The Birth of the Prison,* tr. Alan Sheridan (New York: Vintage, 1979), pp. 45–46.

p. 114, applies more or less to the skyscraper: Janet Semple, *Bentham's Prison: A Study of the Panopticon Penitentiary* (Oxford: Clarendon Press, 1993), p. 116.

p. 114, "deprived of the most basic privacy": Semple, *Bentham's Prison,* p. 128.

p. 115, themselves the event: Robin Evans, *The Fabrication of Virtue: English Prison Architecture, 1750–1840* (Cambridge, England: Cambridge University Press, 1982), p. 209.

p. 115, "standing a great chance to be so": Bentham, *Works,* IV, 40, 44.

p. 115, by an omniscient God: Hannah Arendt, *Lectures on Kant's Political Philosophy* (Chicago: University of Chicago Press, 1982), pp. 49–50.

p. 115, the "invisible omnipresence" of a deity: John Dinwiddy, *Bentham* (Oxford: Oxford University Press, 1989), p. 92.

p. 116, "a simple idea in Architecture!": Bentham, *Works,* IV, 39.

p. 116, "anarchical fallacies" of the French Revolution: Bentham, *Works,* X, 572; J. H. Burns, "Bentham and the French Revolution," *Transactions of the Royal Historical Society,* series 5, 16 (1966): 95–114.

p. 116, "the dictates of reason alone": Evans, *Fabrication of Virtue,* p. 198.

p. 116, "colour, perfume, and lights": Semple, *Bentham's Prison,* p. 296.

p. 117, "other people's projects, intentions, and desires": Alasdair MacIntyre, *After Virtue: A Study in Moral Theory* (Notre Dame: University of Notre Dame Press, 1981), p. 99.

p. 117, "clear and unambiguously legible meaning": Maza, *Private Lives and Public Affairs,* p. 66.

p. 117, "a passive object on which he can act": Gary Saul Morson, "Prosaic Bakhtin: *Landmarks,* Anti-Intelligentsialism and the Russian Counter-Tradition," *Common Knowledge* 2 (Spring 1993): 65.

p. 118, "the Public-Opinion Tribunal": Bentham, *Works,* IX, 86.

p. 118, "assurance of not being observed": Bentham, *Works,* IV, 86.

p. 118, paranoid detail of his *Constitutional Code*: Bentham even prescribes the position of a judge's bed: *Works,* IX, 542n.

p. 119, "predictive practices of others": MacIntyre, *After Virtue,* p. 99.

p. 120, "To be so easily seen through I am afraid is pitiful": Elizabeth Bennet; Austen, *Complete Novels,* p. 255.

p. 120, "a perfect right to despise him": Dostoevsky, *The Brothers Karamazov,* p. 587.

p. 120, "all windows, skylights, and tubular furniture": Broyard, *Intoxicated by My Illness,* p. 21.

p. 121, "millions at a time": Cited in David Spadafora, *The Idea of Progress in Eighteenth-Century Britain* (New Haven: Yale University Press, 1990), p. 178.

p. 122, "They live in the full view of all": Thomas More, *Utopia,* tr. Robert M. Adams (New York: Norton, 1975), p. 49.

p. 122, it is in the utopian tradition that Bentham's Panopticon is rooted: Semple, *Bentham's Prison,* ch. 12.

p. 122, "actually looked at and transformed the dead part of her": Buchholz, *Live Longer, Live Larger,* p. 282.

Calculation versus Judgment

p. 125, sometimes the clinician: Sherwin Nuland, *New Republic,* September 18, 2000.

p. 127, to ponder that twenty-three-point difference: *New Republic,* April 1, 1996.

p. 127, "its ability to learn from it": Hannah Arendt, *Crises of the Republic* (New York: Harcourt Brace Jovanovich, 1972), pp. 37, 39.

p. 130, "sexual activity might be causally involved in risk": Greaves, *Cancer,* p. 165. On eunuchs and prostate cancer, see p. 163.

Calculation, Birth, Death

p. 132, "replicas; that is, children": Rabelais, *Gargantua and Pantagruel,* tr. J. M. Cohen (Harmondsworth, Middlesex: Penguin, 1955), pp. 298, 300, 301.

p. 132, the continuation of their own being: "Among the gifts, graces, and prerogatives which the Sovereign Creator, God Almighty, endowed and embellished human nature in the beginning, one seems to me to stand alone, and to excell all others; that is the one by which we can, in this mortal state, acquire a kind of immortality and, in the course of this transitory life, perpetuate our name and seed; which we do by lineage sprung from us in lawful marriage" (p. 193).

p. 133, "could you bear to part with me?": Cited in Dinwiddy, *Bentham,* pp. 6–7.

p. 133, "called third parties into existence": John Stuart Mill, *On Liberty* (New York: Norton, 1975), p. 96.

p. 134, "other sisters and brothers [were] successively added": John Stuart Mill, *Autobiography* (Indianapolis: Library of Liberal Arts, 1957), p. 8.

p. 134, "a life or lives of wretchedness and depravity to the offspring": Mill, *On Liberty,* p. 100.

p. 134, "whether our society should reproduce itself at all": Christopher Lasch, *The Culture of Narcissism* (New York: Warner, 1979), p. 357.

p. 135, with the purpose of "doing away" with them: Taylor, *Sources of the Self,* p. 159.

p. 135, "accept death proudly and serenely like a god": Dostoevsky, *The Brothers Karamazov,* p. 789.

p. 135, "survived significantly longer than women who didn't attend": Bostwick, MacLennan, and Larson, *Prostate Cancer,* pp. 228–229.

p. 136, "a potion which puts them painlessly to sleep": More, *Utopia,* p. 65.

p. 136, nor is his decision to die authorized by any priest. The administration of the last rites, some time before, is portrayed as a sham.

p. 136, a term of social policy: Sherwin Nuland, *New Republic,* May 27, 2002.

The Death of Ivan Ilych: The Limits of Knowledge

p. 138, "keeps her processes absolutely unknown": Montaigne, p. 400.

p. 138, "a warning to the living": Tolstoy, *Short Fiction,* p. 125.

p. 138, if things had taken another turn: Gary Saul Morson, *Narrative and Freedom: The Shadows of Time* (New Haven: Yale University Press, 1994).

p. 139, "the pervasive role of chance": Greaves, *Cancer,* p. 21.

p. 141, "the small concerns of this world": Lionel Trilling, *The Opposing Self* (New York: Viking, 1995), p. 163.

p. 147, "violate any regulating norms which might be thrust upon him": M. M. Bakhtin, *Problems of Dostoevsky's Poetics,* tr. Caryl Emerson (Minneapolis: University of Minnesota Press, 1984), p. 59.

p. 149, "Rousseau's noble savage": Isaiah Berlin, *Russian Thinkers* (Harmondsworth, Middlesex: Penguin, 1978), p. 53.

p. 149, "never to profit in any way by the death of anyone dear to me": Rousseau, *Confessions,* p. 572.

p. 151, "They are process, not product": Morson, *Narrative and Freedom,* p. 172.

p. 151, "Contingency always reigns": Morson, *Narrative and Freedom,* p. 172.

p. 152, "giving time for the improbable to happen": Greaves, *Cancer,* p. 217.

p. 153, "had spent the best years of their lives on that business": Tolstoy, *War and Peace*, p. 700. Cf. the portrayal of the medical specialist called in to examine Kitty at the beginning of Part Two of *Anna Karenina*.

p. 154, "prevent you from imagining yourself free of cancer": Buchholz, *Live Longer, Live Larger*, p. 32.

Small Offices of Kindness

p. 155, "the anxious avaricious tentacles of the self": Murdoch, *Sovereignty of Good*, p. 101.

p. 156, "as if in readiness for what he had to do next": Tolstoy, *Short Fiction*, pp. 125, 129.

p. 157, "can see other things as they are": Murdoch, *Sovereignty of Good*, p. 101.

p. 158, too angry to experience gratitude: Ehrenreich, "Welcome to Cancerland."

Cruel Choices

p. 160, "the revelatory power of the extraordinary": Michael André Bernstein, *New Republic*, September 27, 1999.

p. 160, "the Rome of the Republic or even of the Antonines": Isaiah Berlin, *The Proper Study of Mankind* (New York: Farrar, Straus and Giroux, 1998), pp. 311–312.

p. 160, Hard choices are things we prefer to evade. In the Wife of Bath's Tale—a sort of Arthurian fairy tale with a difference—a knight is given a brutally hard choice between having a fair but possibly unfaithful wife and an ugly but faithful one. In the end he receives a wife both fair and faithful.

p. 161, "the reconciling and combining of opposites": Mill, *On Liberty*, p. 46.

p. 162, the "rise" of one thing spells the "fall" of another": Hirschman, *Rhetoric of Reaction*, p. 121.

p. 162, "I *could* have it both ways": Milken's Introduction to a cookbook by Beth Ginsberg, available on his website.

p. 162, "the quality of our usual attachments": Murdoch, *Sovereignty of Good*, p. 89.

p. 162, "still lead a full and satisfying life": Bostwick, MacLennan, and Larson, *Prostate Cancer*, p. 240.

p. 163, "powerful, passionate, and sexy": Bostwick, MacLennan, and Larson, *Prostate Cancer,* p. 221.

p. 164, when people possessed of an archaic mentality supposed that choices had costs. A hard choice: a woman's decision whether or not to take estrogen, thereby increasing her risk of breast cancer but decreasing the risk of heart disease, osteoporosis, and endometrial cancer.

p. 164, "catching them early is our only hope": Shannon Brownlee, *New Republic,* April 22, 2002.

p. 165, "an attempt to *make* him answer it in a particular way": R. M. Hare, *The Language of Morals* (Oxford: Oxford University Press, 1964), p. 15.

p. 165, "the informed choices available to the rest of us": Greaves, *Cancer,* p. 260.

p. 166, "a healthy state of political life": Mill, *On Liberty,* p. 46.

Publicity and Enlightenment

p. 167, "And 'publicity' appeared": Cited in John Christian Laursen, "The Subversive Kant: The Vocabulary of 'Public' and 'Publicity,'" *Political Theory* 14 (1986): 594.

p. 167, "each unhealthy organism is unhealthy in its own way": Gary Saul Morson, *Hidden in Plain View: Narrative and Creative Potentials in 'War and Peace'* (Stanford: Stanford University Press, 1987), p. 172.

p. 167, "disorders of cell and tissue function": Greaves, *Cancer,* p. 3.

p 168, physics envy: Hirschman, *Rhetoric of Reaction,* p. 155.

p. 169, "medicine for the individual and for society": Peter Gay, *The Enlightenment: An Interpretation,* Vol. 2: *The Science of Freedom* (New York: Alfred A. Knopf, 1969), pp. 13, 16, 17.

p. 169, in the vanguard of the campaign for progress: Isaac Kramnick, *Republicanism and Bourgeois Radicalism: Political Ideology in Late Eighteenth-Century England and America* (Ithaca: Cornell University Press, 1990), p. 93.

p. 169, "an act of great philanthropy": Flaubert, *Madame Bovary,* tr. Mildred Marmur (New York: Signet, 1964), p. 176.

p. 170, "the authority of parents, priests, and lawgivers": Lasch, *Haven in a Heartless World,* p. 100.

p. 170, "no evil can continue": Bentham, *Works,* II, 314.

p. 170, "the medicalization of religion": Lasch, *Haven in a Heartless World,* p. 98.

p. 171, "before it can be cured": Martin Luther King, Jr., *Why We Can't Wait* (New York: Harper and Row, 1964), p. 88.

p. 171, "has to be capable of being made public": Bok, *Lying,* p. 97.

p. 172, "ministerial cabinets and royal councils": Maza, *Private Lives and Public Affairs,* p. 64. In the minds of the revolutionaries, accordingly, the pomp of the old regime and its secret diplomatic practices were two facets of the same corruption, and the refashioners of French diplomacy sought to purge it of both secrecy and excessive show. Linda Frey and Marsha Frey, "'The Reign of the Charlatans is Over': The French Revolutionary Attack on Diplomatic Practice," *Journal of Modern History* 65 (1993): 706–744.

p. 173, as Kant himself did: Kant, "The Contest of Faculties," in *Political Writings,* tr. H. B. Nisbet (Cambridge, England: Cambridge University Press, 1992), p. 186.

p. 173, the opening up of the political system to the light of publicity: Maza, *Private Lives and Public Affairs,* p. 114.

p. 173, more or less secret even in eighteenth-century America: Michael Schudson, "Was There Ever a Public Sphere? If So, Where? Reflections on the American Case," in *Habermas and the Public Sphere,* ed. Craig Calhoun (Cambridge, Mass.: MIT, 1993), pp. 154–155. In England, parliamentary debate was technically, but only technically, secret. See Dror Wahrman, "Virtual Representation: Parliamentary Reporting and the Languages of Class in the 1790s," *Past and Present* No. 136 (1992): 86.

p. 173, literate, propertied men who spoke in the name of the general good: Habermas, *Structural Transformation of the Public Sphere,* p. 52.

p. 174, influenced by the ideals of the American Revolution in the first place: On the international public of the later eighteenth century, see Marilyn Butler, *Romantics, Rebels and Reactionaries: English Literature and Its Background 1760–1830* (Oxford: Oxford University Press, 1981), pp. 15–16.

p. 174, moral action must be consistent with being made public: Jefferson, similarly, came to believe that the most effectual way to preserve laws and cultural documents was not to secret them away by means of "vaults and locks" but to publish them. See Eisenstein, *Printing Revolution in Early Modern Europe,* p. 81.

p. 174, "he liked to have the gods as witnesses to his actions": Cited in Starobinski, *Transparency and Obstruction,* p. 11.

p. 175, "Every body is eager to look at him": Smith, *Theory of Moral Sentiments,* p. 51.

p. 175, "the corruption of our moral sentiments": Smith, *Theory of Moral Sentiments,* p. 61. Wordsworth offers the Lyrical Ballads, with their "common" language and subjects, as an antidote to the depravity of public taste.

p. 175, "the displays of power and exhibitions of art": Maza, *Private Lives and Public Affairs,* p. 11. On public opinion as a tribunal of the written word, see William Hazlitt, *Selected Writings* (Oxford: Oxford University Press, 1991), p. 89: "Let all the wrongs public and private produced in France by arbitrary power and exclusive privileges for a thousand years be collected in a volume, and let this volume be read by all who have hearts to feel or capacity to understand, and the strong, stifling sense of oppression and kindling burst of indignation that would follow would be that impulse of public opinion that led to the French Revolution."

p. 176, "oriented around . . . printed texts": Joan Landes, *Women and the Public Sphere in the Age of the French Revolution* (Ithaca: Cornell University Press, 1988), pp. 40–41.

p. 176, "a public in the truest sense of the word": Kant, "An Answer to the Question: 'What Is Enlightenment?'" in *Political Writings,* p. 56.

p. 176, "the sign and guarantee of liberty": Lynn Hunt, *Politics, Culture, and Class in the French Revolution* (Berkeley: University of California Press, 1984), p. 74.

p. 176, the intimacy of a conspiracy: Arendt, *Lectures on Kant's Political Philosophy,* p. 60. Cf. Eisenstein, *Printing Revolution in Early Modern Europe,* p. 95: "To hear an address delivered, people have to come together; to read a printed report encourages individuals to draw apart. 'What the orators of Rome and Athens were in the midst of a people *assembled,*' said Malesherbes in an address of 1775, 'men of letters are in the midst of a *dispersed* people.'"

p. 176, "to expose it to daylight in all of its ugliness": Cited in Maza, *Private Lives and Public Affairs,* p. 118.

p. 177, a punishment in front of the crowd: Cited in R. M. Wiles, "Crowd-Pleasing Spectacles in Eighteenth-Century England," *Journal of Popular Culture* 1 (1967–1968): 93.

p. 177, "the feeble influence of reason and religion over the human mind": Cited in Foucault, *Discipline and Punish,* p. 10.

p. 178, "the gibbet and the hulks": Cited in Daniel C. Hallin, "The American News Media: A Critical Theory Perspective," in *Critical Theory and Public Life,* ed. John Forester (Cambridge, Mass.: MIT Press, 1988), p. 132. Gibbet and hulks figure powerfully in Dickens's *Great Expectations.*

p. 178, as if one form of publicity were being advocated in another's place: The passage from the tradition of cruel spectacles to the therapeutic culture of modernity has been recounted by Foucault in *Discipline and Punish*. In the last and greatest work by the novelist of punishment, Dostoevsky, the mechanisms of enlightenment discussed by Foucault—expert opinions, dissections of the soul, reformed legal procedures—are focused on a "criminal" who didn't commit the crime, who still lives traditions like dueling, and who little believes in the fashion of journalism that has made him a sensation across Russia.

p. 178, "no legal existence": John Money, *Experience and Identity: Birmingham and the West Midlands, 1760–1800* (Montreal: McGill-Queen's University Press, 1977), pp. 39–40.

p. 179, "no evil can continue": Bentham, *Works*, II, 314.

p. 180, "gigantic secret societies that . . . spanned the Atlantic": Wood, "Conspiracy and the Paranoid Style," p. 407.

The Public and the Private

p. 184, "I need a chamber-pot every minute": *The Heart of Boswell*, ed. Mark Harris (New York: McGraw-Hill, 1981), p. 152.

p. 185, "understating your suffering": Montaigne, p. 396.

p. 186, "which occurred on February 4th of this year 1882": Tolstoy, *Short Fiction*, p. 123.

p. 187, "this deceptive, but clear and always flattering presentation": Tolstoy, *War and Peace*, pp. 1310–1311. The exchange of doubts for deceptions takes place, too, in *The Death of Ivan Ilych*, "the general opinion" becoming public opinion ("I was going up in public opinion, but to the same extent life was ebbing away from me") and official lies "a terrible and huge deception which had hidden both life and death."

p. 187, "both possibilities are always present, as they are in life": Morson, *Narrative and Freedom*, p. 159.

p. 188, "formulate a coherent scheme of what they do": Frye, *Anatomy of Criticism*, p. 229.

p. 188, "it certainly didn't apply to himself": Tolstoy, *Short Fiction*, p. 149. Seeing that Kiesewetter is identified as "a follower of Kant," we can say that Kiesewetter's Law satirizes at one remove the sort of legalism so pronounced in Kant, as when he asks whether the principle of an action can be made into a universal law.

p. 189, "all the selfishness of imaginary complaints": Austen, *Complete Novels,* p. 1000.

p. 190, "the launch of Paxil as an anti-shyness agent was a media event": Healy, "Good Science or Good Business?" p. 20.

A Stone Without a Cherry

p. 193, "the seedcake warm and chewed": James Joyce, *Ulysses* (Oxford: Oxford University Press, 1993), p. 167.

p. 193, "an antecedent Power or Principle in the Seed": Coleridge, cited in M. H. Abrams, *The Mirror and the Lamp* (Oxford: Oxford University Press, 1953), p. 171.

INDEX

Arendt, Hannah, 82, 95, 127
Aristotle, 145–148
Austen, Jane, 27–28, 30, 54, 56, 70, 120, 188–189

Bentham, Jeremy, 38, 56–57, 93, 108–123, 124, 131, 133, 168, 170, 179
Berlin, Isaiah, 56, 160
Bernays, Edward, 62
Bernstein, Michael André, 26, 160
Boccaccio, 83
Bok, Sissela, 3–7, 9, 19, 21–22, 171, 174
Brachytherapy, 11, 24, 46, 105–107, 120–121, 125, 183, 191
Breast cancer, xii, xv, 22, 31, 37, 46–53, 56, 58–59, 61–68, 101, 112, 164
Broyard, Anatole, 110, 120
Brueghel, Peter, 24–33, 70, 93, 155
Buber, Martin, 170

Carlyle, Thomas, 110, 112, 125
Chaucer, 8, 15, 32

A NOTE ON THE AUTHOR

Stewart Justman was born in New York City and studied at Columbia University. Since the 1970s he has lived in Missoula, Montana, where he is professor of English at the University of Montana. He has also written *The Springs of Liberty* and *The Psychological Mystique*. He is married with two children.